Praise for *Conspiracies of Kindness*

"Pssst! a little secret: The most influential force in our world is not power but compassion, empathy, and love. *Conspiracies of Kindness* by Michael Ortiz Hill shows why. Handle with care: This luminous book can change your life."
— Larry Dossey, MD
Author of *The Power Of Premonitions*

"Brimming with insights, alive with stories that anchor them in your heart, this banquet of a book shows that compassionate presence is ever and always a choice we can make. And we can make it over and over again. Fresh, unpredictable, and uncontrived."

— Joanna Macy, author *World as Lover, World as Self.*

"This book is a marvelous revelation... Michael builds upon his experiences in nursing to provide rich teaching tales from the everyday work of a hospital that point us toward love and kindness. I recommend this book most highly as an engaging and uplifting read that's both inspirational and educational – perfect for both the beach and the classroom setting in health sciences and anthropology."

— Lewis Mehl-Madrona, MD, Ph.D., author of *Coyote Medicine*

"This book is an invitation to enter the territory of the boundless heart. Rich in from-the-soul- stories, and rooted in deep recognition of our human kinship, [It] has much to teach us about healing, living, and loving."
— Aura Glaser, author of *A Call to Compassion*

"Chock full of beautiful, elegant wisdom... truly a magnificent piece of work. It resonates with heart, depth and the humility of real experience. It is a gift to us all."
— Dr. David Forbes, MD
President of the American Holistic Medicine Association

"This book invites a deeper level of the work of caring. I hope it will reach as many practitioners as possible."
— Jean Watson Ph.D. RN.
Author of *Nursing: The Philosophy and Science of Caring*

"Drawing on his own struggles with the mysterious microbial demons of MS and a range of fascinating encounters with patients and doctors, Michael Ortiz Hill gives us a soul-stirring meditation on the nature of illness, life and death. Reading these stories on the healing qualities of compassion, you feel empowered and encouraged on your own journey toward wholeness." — Ralph Metzner, Ph.D.

Author of *The Well of Remembrance* and *The Unfolding Self.*

"Michael Ortiz Hill is truly a alchemist. Patient care experiences that are often perceived by direct care providers as lead in Craft of Compassion are illuminated as golden opportunities and should motivate all nurses to live compassion. Once his message is swallowed and absorbed the effect is powerful." — Lisa Speer, RN

"Michael Ortiz Hill never fails to capture you, reaching deep into your heart and "soul," stirring thoughts and emotions that ultimately bring peace of spirit. Absorb his words in *Conspiracies of Kindness.* "

— Mary Horan RN, MN

"Michael is a gifted teacher, and the lessons from this book have deeply enriched my work as a family medicine physician. The idea that compassion is a teachable craft with skills to be practiced brings it from the mystical into the daily world, which of course is where we all need it. I recommend this book to anyone involved in caring for the ill."

— Kjersten Gmeiner, MD

"This book is for those who have hit bottom and know it. Michael Ortiz Hill tells stories about the most difficult cases in health care, the worst situations that burn out those who care and break their hearts. Then he shows how things can be made better. There isn't always an immediate or even long-term happy ending, but there's something worth calling hope. For those who need it, [this book] can bring life. For health care, Hill opens a space to begin again." — Arthur W. Frank

author of *At the Will of the Body* and *Letting Stories Breathe.*

"Burdens of life transform into magical opportunities to expand your Soul's power within the ocean of compassion and kindness when confronted by the devastations and miracles of our human existence. This is what our guide, Michael Ortiz Hill, shows us as we travel the paths of human sorrow and resurrections in *Conspiracies of Kindness.*"

— Dr. Carol Francis, *Make Life Happen*

2

Conspiracies of Kindness

The Craft of Compassion at the Bedside of the Ill

Michael Ortiz Hill

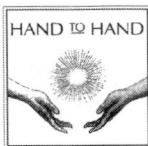

HAND TO HAND

Hand to Hand is a community based endeavor that supports independently published works and public events, free of the restrictions that arise from commercial and political concerns. It is a forum for artists who are in dynamic and reciprocal relationship with their communities for the sake of peacemaking, restoring culture and the planet. For further information regarding **Hand to Hand** please write to us at: P.O. Box 186, Topanga, CA, 90290, USA. Or visit us on the web at:

www.handtohandpublishing.com

Hand to Hand First Edition, November, 2010
05 04 03 02 01

ISBN: 978-0-9720718-6-4

Book and Cover Design: Stephan David Hewitt
Cover Photo by: Richard Grossman

For more information about special discounts for bulk purchases, please contact:

> Hand to Hand Publishing
> PO Box 186
> Topanga, CA 90290

Contents

16. The Illness Runs through Everybody,

Conversation with Robert Carroll, MD

17. Beatitude, Death, and the Mother of Beauty

Step Three: Radical Empathy

18. Idiot Compassion

19. Narcissism Devours Presence

20. La Familia and Radical Empathy

21. The Kindest of Buddhas

22. Surviving Something No One Should Survive

Step Four: Living Compassion

23. Kindness Is a Spirit

24. Love is the Only Medicine I Know

25. Without Thinking About Compassion, It Flows – *Conversation with Jalaladin Ebrahim*

26. Awakening to Who You Have Become

27. The Presence of the Everyday

Conversation with Katherine Brown-Saltzman, RN

28. The Serenity Prayer and the Three Faces of Living Compassion

Conclusion : The Best You Can Ever Do

6

For my father, Milford Hill (1925-1977),

my mother, Adelina Ortiz de Hill,

and my wife, Deena Metzger,

that what you planted in me may blossom.

For my grandson Shylo Lockwood who was born smiling.

Welcome to the home planet, little one.

We are put on earth but a little space

That we might learn to bear the beams of love.

— *William Blake*

Love as much as you can from where you are with what you've got.
That's the best you can ever do.
Remember, it's the process, not the content that counts.

— *Cheri Huber*

Work is love made visible.

— *Ama Ata Aidoo*

In the middle of nursing duties and dirty beds and bloody bandages there is magic. Where there is pain and fear and loneliness, there are miracles. In the small hours of the night when there are dying and dark things, there is light.

— *Carolyn Parnal Fink, RN*

Preface

A fundamental theme in this book is the transformation of suffering into compassion. I was instructed in this teaching as a young man. My parents separated when I was eleven, and my father had his first major heart attack three months later. I came of age watching his slow-motion suicide. Liquor and cigarettes. There wasn't a thing I could do to save him.

At the same time that he descended into his dark night of the soul, I slipped into my own. For three years I lived as a homeless teenager in Santa Cruz, California. My life was gathering garbage to eat, sleeping under the freeway bridge if it rained, solitude, dysentery, lice, scabies, and an extreme psyche. But also reading, prayer, and meditation. I had dropped out of high school, thank God, and was getting a real education.

Even during those years as a homeless teenager I would visit my father in Southern California every few months. He was my first spiritual teacher and my first partner in intellectual dialogue. He taught me to meditate when I was sixteen. I was a creature of his library: Buddhism, Jung, Thomas Merton, St. John of the Cross, Sri Aurobindo, Alan Watts, and Herman Hesse. Aldous Huxley's *Perennial Philosophy* engrossed me because it was about the common language shared between spiritual traditions, and clearly the ethos of lovingkindness was pervasive.

In the room in which my father meditated stood an icon of Kwan Yin, the Buddhist goddess of compassion, that he won in a card game in Korea during the war. Being raised Catholic, I took her to be the equivalent of the Blessed Virgin Mary. "Some are taken by miracles like walking on water, but the real miracle is compassion and it's available to everybody. Live by that, Michael," my father told me.

At one point when I thought I was going mad, I called my father and spoke to him of ecstasy and terror. He listened deeply and said, "I know it's frightening, but it's a rite of initiation and you can trust it. I went through the same thing when I was your age."

He had been cracked open as a teenager when his uncle was shot over a poker game in Cloudcroft, New Mexico. We both learned early in life about how damned difficult it is to be human and that the circumstances of this life are a school for learning compassion.

My father was a profound man and profoundly broken. Radiantly imperfect. His slow suicide was swift enough. It took him all of nine years to find death.

In August, 1977, the night before I returned to Santa Cruz, I burst into tears and told him, "I think you are dying." The next morning, a week before he died, he dropped me off at a freeway onramp to hitchhike four hundred miles home. There was a lack of grace between us, a clumsiness.

"God bless you," were his last words.

"God bless you too, dad."

Dylan Thomas writes, "After the first death there is no other." I know that to be true. When my father died he left behind the mystery of death and grief as a gift. That mystery has shaped my life. Suffering transforms into compassion if you're attentive.

My mother, Adelina Ortiz de Hill, was a medical social worker when my father died and was much involved in the then-nascent hospice movement. Intrigued by her stories and wanting to understand death, I volunteered to work with the dying myself. This led to my training to become an RN.

Hospice was the crucible in which I invented myself. With my hospice patients I envisioned and re-visioned who I might have been if I had been at my father's bedside when he passed.

It was in hospice that I began to imagine the craft of compassion that I would later apply to nursing. My father's death became the ground for learning solidarity with others who are afflicted. Over the years, that ground became more trustworthy with everyone I've cared for. As much as I was undone by my father's death, grief and commitment to the ill has made it possible to carry his teaching forward.

I am now at the age my father was when he told his kid: "It's a rite of initiation and you can trust it." With those words he stepped forth into a new role of elder, and now it is my time to step forth.

Young as he was, he said exactly the right thing.

Young as I am, may I speak honorably of what I have learned.

Acknowledgments

This book - like most everything I've ever written - found its genesis with my wife, Deena Metzger. Many of the stories I tell here I first told to Deena, soaking away a work week in a tub together and catching up on the odyssey of our days apart. "You must write a book about this, Mr. Ortizy."

The emphatic **MUST** was underscored by my multiple sclerosis diagnosis and indeed the first of perhaps fifty drafts of this work was written during a couple of months of solitude and meditation when I gave over the fierce and kind Guest of MS.

The miracle of being healed is inscribed between the words of *Conspiracies*.

Gratitude to Deena and the incomparable Lady of Solitude.

Intimacy with these two has made me the person that I am.

Twenty years ago, Deena and I were lost in the rainforest of Monteverde, Costa Rica, after nightfall. To the jaguars that come out to hunt in the dark we would, no doubt, be delicious. Fireflies came and, one by one, flashed green - then disappeared. These little one made it possible to discern the trail out of the bush. They saved our lives.

I've privately called my editor, Carol Bond, the shaman of the fireflies. Lost in the dark night of Conspiracies, her comments lit the trail for a couple of years. I'm indebted to Carol for the refinement of the four steps that frame this book and my workshops on the Craft of Compassion.

Gratitude upon gratitude to Stephan Hewitt who polished this final of final drafts and kept faith with the music of it.

Homage also to Sharron Dorr of Quest books for believing in me and Dr Carol Francis and her exquisite openness as an interviewer. Carol fed the proverbial fire under my ass and received this book under her imprint, Make Life Happens.

Gratitude to Dr.s Bill Manahan and David Forbes - respectively the past and present presidents of the American Holistic Medical Association. Bill and David both live by the ethos "first, do no harm" but further than that they know that compassion is the heart and soul of medicine. It is an honor to break bread with such.

Gratitude to Aura Glaser who received this book most gracefully. I was intimidated connecting with Aura as this book relies on a redefinition of the quintessence section of her book, The Call to Compassion. Our dialogues on the common ground between us - both inspired by the lack of compassion being taught in our professional training - was most illuminating.

My mother lives alone in a cabin her father built in the Sangre de Cristo mountains outside of Santa Fe. When I asked her what was the spiritual choice that she'd want to die alone she answered with the Spanish folk saying:

El viejo árbol muere de pie.
(The old tree dies on its feet.)

My mother is in her eighties now and has congestive heart failure like my father. When I say gratitude to Adelina Ortiz de Hill of course I speak of the reciprocation of gift giving. This book is, as much as anything, a gift to her. What you have planted may I bring to fruition.

I call Dr. Kjersten Gmeiner, Fringer. Kjersten and I teach the Craft together and the running joke between us is - she being an MD of the feminine persuasion and I being a male RN - who is the Fred and who is the Ginger between us? "I CAN'T dance backwards in high heels!" complained Kjersten.
"What - you think *I* can?" I'd retort.

As a coconspirator of kindness, Kjersten is peerless.

Finally the birth of this book coincides with the birth of my grandson, Shylo Lockwood. Shylo was born smiling and his smile blesses us all.

This book was written for the future.

About the Cover

The origami cranes that grace the cover of this book were made by Mrs. Yasu, a Japanese woman living in a nursing home. Mrs. Yasu learned to make origami as a young girl in Tokyo from her grandmother and her sister. When she lost her eyesight in 1996, she also went into the darkness of spiritual doubt. At first she thought that if she made a thousand cranes for God her eyesight would be given her back. Later her prayer became: "Just your will." Eventually she discovered that she could pray over the cranes as gifts for others who suffer.

Her husband died in 2004, and since then she has lived in a nursing home, rarely leaving her room. "I can make twenty-five cranes a day, but with my arthritis it is sometimes very hard, very painful. When I make them, I pray that I follow God in everything that I do."

I read her chapter 14 of this book, about her ministry of the cranes, and she gave me fifteen-hundred cranes for my patients. I also asked if I could use a picture of the cranes for the cover of this book. She smiled: "*Arigato* – thank you very much."

Introduction: The Heart of the Matter

This book is written for anyone who takes the matter of compassion seriously. In such a time as we live, I dare say nothing is more important. Simple-minded and stubborn, this book proposes that compassion is a craft and thus can be learned and practiced like cultivating crops or raising animals. The refinement of compassion, like any true craft, is a life's work.

Dr. Jean Watson. Ph.D., RN, writes in *Nursing: The Philosophy and Science of Caring*, "Of the many problems that can arise in nursing, perhaps one of the most common is the failure to establish rapport, being insensitive, unable to connect or create an alliance with another. Put another way, a major problem is the lack of reflective, mindful awareness of how one's presence and consciousness toward self and others can and do affect the nature and outcome of one's relationship with another, whether the other is a colleague, a patient, or a family member."

The transition to caring for the ill is as fierce as any tribal rite of initiation, though few speak of it as such. From listening to the stories of doctors and nurses, three intertwining themes emerge that define the struggle to keep the heart open.

First, there is staggering within the reality of suffering, the sheer mass of unanswerable needs. How does one sift through overwhelm and find the person of the other, as well the presence of oneself? How does one gracefully discern what can be given and what cannot? What is the place of kindness and generosity towards oneself?

Second, there is the specific shape of oneself, one's wounds, one's fears of giving and receiving compassion. Many of us were told as children and in our professional training not to feel too much. Clinical distance was praised as professionalism. Watson, on the other hand, writes that "authentic connection and responses are necessary as an ethic: the authenticity of the self reveals the integrity of the professional."

Relationship-based caring, a new and ancient shift of paradigm that is beginning to reawaken the soul of medicine, is fundamental to this book. Ivan Illich writes of the change in the nineteenth century when that relationship was severed – we no longer treated people suffering from this or that, we treated diseases. Every healthcare provider and every patient knows the bitter alienation of this, and this book celebrates the in-breaking of another way of seeing.

Last, as Aldous Huxley wrote in *The Perennial Philosophy*, the institutions of the modern world are based on "organized lovelessness." Thus again the severing and reestablishing of relationship. Every healthcare provider has experienced the systemic crushing of the compassionate impulse if only through something as brutal yet ordinary as understaffing. The heart closes when one is in a hurry.

These three coexisting realities form the threshold in our training and our day to day work that we must cross to meet the heart of compassion.

Birth, chronic illness, death, the extremities of fear, pain, and madness – healthcare engages the most fundamental realities of being human and therefore the essential questions that we must ask ourselves in order to live fully.

Compassion is a vast subject and to grasp it as a learnable craft it helps to break it down into a set of steps. When we begin taking steps we rightly feel we are going somewhere and intuit correctly that many have walked this path before us.

What I am calling the four steps of compassion are drawn from the work of the spiritual teacher, Dr. Aura Glaser. Glaser noticed in her training as a psychotherapist that compassion was not taught. I was drawn to Glaser's reflections because in the training of medical personnel there is a hollowness since compassion is likewise not taught. She comments in her book, *A Call to Compassion: Bringing Buddhist Practices of the Heart into the Soul of Psychotherapy*, "the Tibetan tradition is replete with instruction and methodology" on compassion because "while the rest of the world was focused on outer progress, Tibet was focused on inner development." Glaser distills four major points from the essential actions and principles of these teachings: compassion for self, compassion for others, exchanging self and other, and no self and no other.

I speak of these four distillations as "steps," and they form the backbone of this book.

The first step – the foundation of compassionate activity and thus of the three steps that follow – is *self-compassion*. Step Two is *compassion toward others*. This is compassion as it is mostly commonly understood and expressed. As such, stories and reflections on compassion for others are the most abundant.

Steps Three and Four grow out of compassion for others. Step Three is *radical empathy*, extending oneself empathically into another's experience. More than the expression of compassion to another being, it is an identification with that being's experience. It is summarized in the Cherokee saying that you don't know another person until you've walked two moons in their moccasins.

Step Four, the fulfillment of the path of compassion, is *living compassion*. Here one's sense of self and also the sense of the other person as an individual fall away, if only for a moment. There is, as Glaser calls it, "no self and no other." Only compassion itself remains.

The first two steps fall within the familiar, personalized paradigm, but with Steps Three and Four, the fixity and centrality of the self begin to loosen. The self slips to the side so compassion with its radiant intelligence can move unimpeded.

At the same time, compassion, being a moment-by-moment practice, is not really about steps. The Steps lead to you the edge of what you know, and you step off that edge into a paradigm shift. So "Steps" demands a caveat. In fact, all four Steps can make up the practice of compassion on any given day. A practitioner may be in any one of these four aspects of compassion at any moment according to what is needed.

In another sense, the four Steps form a circle. Living compassion circles back to the "self" of self-compassion, but in a deeper way. Not I, ego, but being present with a kind of transparency to one's core nature – what some traditions call soul or the ground of being. Compassion, the Buddhists say, is our "original nature," and though we forever muddy this ordinary truth, it is nonetheless always present. We need to simply pause and open our eyes to know it.

This book progresses through the interplay of reflections and stories, many of them my own, some gathered from others. The names of the ill have been changed to protect the privacy of individuals.

The book also includes interviews with other healthcare practitioners, who offer their own perspectives on the practice and experience of compassion. Their names have not been changed. They are "elders," people who have walked the path of compassion long enough to act with depth and directness. They are not unique. No doubt elders of their caliber walk the halls of healthcare facilities across the country. Their colleagues and patients know them.

It's probably no accident that many of the interviewees in this book have a religious tradition in which they ground their practice of compassion. When a spiritual life is practiced for real, in genuine relation to teachings on compassion, there can be a profound perspective to step outside oneself and relate to a suffering person. I intentionally chose interviewees from different monotheistic traditions because these are the traditions that have largely shaped the world we live in. And also because we do not listen and learn from one another, are swift to judge and we are swift to even make war.

Compassion, rightly understood, is a common language among religion traditions and also between secular and religious people. It's better to join together and conspire to express compassion than to fight each other. Compassion is a practice and a way of life where we can meet and face suffering together.

Krishnamurti said that "truth is a pathless land."

Follow the path together and then step over into the mystery of what cannot be thought or written.

This is the conspiracy of kindness in which human beings can collaborate to sustain the world.

To begin this book, two related premises must be laid out: Compassion is a craft and the foundation of the craft is self-compassion.

As a craft, compassion is learnable and in learning it one is transformed. One learns to drop the self-involvement that snares the activity of compassion. One's feeling life becomes translucent and responsive when one learns to truly meet another. There are ways to convey to someone that they are met and to extend hospitality to a stranger from another culture. To hasten slowly, to pause, and be mindful whatever the rush. These things are learnable, and much of this book is about the particulars of the craft.

Being compassionate toward oneself is the ground of everything.

"Do not build your house upon sand," admonished Jesus. To enter into the spiritual practice of compassion without self-compassion is unsustainable and bears the seeds of frustration and burnout. The joy and meaning of compassion will forever elude you. The Judeo-Muslim-Christian teaching to love your neighbor as yourself requires that you love yourself.

Do unto yourself as you would have others do unto you.

Steven Levine, a spiritual teacher involved in the care of the dying, wrote a book on living each year as one's last. I entered into the "death metaphor" when I was a young hospice volunteer and kept faith with it for a number of years. During those years of "dying" I did not indulge unfinished business with anybody and I began in earnest to pare away self-deception. This was a time of self-clarification.

Getting real with oneself is the most profound act of self-nourishment.

"Know thyself" is the mantra of self-compassion. In coming to make my own acquaintance, I was struck by the obvious: I am neither perfect nor perfectible. Not being perfect took no great insight, but it took a bit to wean from the idea of perfectibility. I came to see the aspiration to be perfect as a stiff variety of narcissism, an altogether cheap imitation of a spiritual life. Wasting my life striving for perfection seemed like the height of folly.

Perfectionism is a cold passion.

There is an honesty that is the edge of ruthless compassion. As Ladner writes, "As compassion entails the wish to free ourselves from suffering, we must see our suffering clearly in order to develop compassion." This honesty involves a holy, and wholly necessary suffering in exposing the self to the self. When I was a young man I would think of my months alone in meditation and prayer as "going naked before God" but of course that was not in the least accurate. When are we ever not naked before God? "The cost of self-deception is your own suffering," says Ladner. The way of self-compassion is really about coming naked before oneself. Difficult, painful and the stuff of great joy. In fact it is the actual path of freedom.

Coming naked seems to be about stripping away, layer by layer, that imposter that pretends to be *me* but actually is my jailer. The habits of narcissism, the three stooges – me, myself and I – forever crave first billing.

Self-compassion is not to be mistaken for selfishness or narcissism. Indeed the fulfillment of self-compassion is full transparency to the presence of another. One cannot be available to another until one is available to oneself with a generous heart.

Getting real with oneself is a relentless act of self love.

All beings know suffering.

And all human beings are required to find their way through the wilderness of suffering, whether their own suffering or that of those they love. Finding their way is what, as much as anything, refines the soul of an adult.

Like refining ore, the refinement and purification of the rough truth of our common experience of suffering can transform it into the simple and direct gesture of compassion. And like refining, the raw stuff of our feeling life, the soul, is remade into elegant ease and forthrightness.

One only needs to be born human to know suffering but healthcare providers especially are tested in this way. For those of us in the healing professions, human suffering is what we are trained to engage with on a daily basis, so we may be more familiar with suffering than most.

When I finished nursing school over twenty years ago, one question insisted on having my attention, and it has persisted ever since: How can the craft of nursing become a practice of compassion?

As a young father and Buddhist who was trying to find his way out of hell – the stink of homeless and the loss of my father – I believed that cultivating compassion was a reliable source of meaning.

I believe compassion is a craft and therefore learnable like nursing. Lovingkindness is a matter of the heart, but it is most certainly also a matter of craft. As a craft it can be learned and refined. This book details the particulars of the craft.

In modern times the idea of craft has been flattened into learning an employable skill. We no longer live in a medieval world where the craft of making a mandolin was passed from father to son, from son to grandson. Yet craft suggests lineage, suggests the possibility of mastery, the full commitment of one's life. It suggests, I believe, even spiritual path and practice.

In *Revisioning Psychology* the archetypal psychologist James Hillman writes of soul-making as a craft. He refers to the ancient Greeks, who believed that the labor of one's hands was also, potentially, the work of making a soul. The Greeks, in turn, likened the making of soul to the making of honey. They observed the diligent bee, chamber by chamber making a honeycomb and in each chamber placing the gathered sweetness. A soul is made, that is, matured, little by little through diligent attention so it can hold substance.

So it is also with compassion as a craft. In responding to the hell of human anguish, nectar is gathered and the soul is shaped to contain it. In this text the nectar is self-compassion, presence for another, the capacity to act skillfully in an ambiguous world, crafting time and hastening slowly, with hospitality, and an eye for beauty.

Ultimately we yield to living compassion.

One tastes this nectar as the activity of compassion nourishes both the giver and the recipient.

Mr. Borges has metastatic cancer and his prognosis is dreadful. He's terrified and in extreme pain. The shift is busy – everyone running around – and his nurse Ellen is swept up in the general urgency. But she's able to remember to pause at Mr. Borges door to let go of the urgency for a few moments so she can "meet" him. Which is to say, listen to his fear while she's injecting a little morphine sulfate into his IV line.

It is in the meeting that compassion happens. Subtle, simple, and direct. Mr. Borges is grateful for the morphine but more so that he was met in his time of uncertainty. "You're the first nurse who took the time to hear me," he said. "Everybody seems so much in a hurry around here. Thank you. Truly."

Ellen responds, "Yes. I apologize. We get very caught up and sometimes forget to be human and pay attention."

She noticed a picture of his daughter on his bedside table – roughly her daughter's age. "We talked of his fear of dying and leaving her fatherless."

What is compassion? In its most simple sense, it is feeling with another.

The word "compassion," from the Latin *com-passio*, means literally "suffering with another." Its close synonym is "sympathy." The root meaning of "passion," despite its other later usages is "suffering," as in the "passion of Christ." Sympathy comes from the Greek *sym-patheia*, literally, "fellow feeling."

When one strips away the cliché and sentimentality that sometimes attach themselves to the word, what is compassion anyway? How does one realize it? What is compassion in truly hopeless circumstances? How does one bring heart to a heartless situation?

Who does the heart shrink from, and what does it mean to step forth to meet that person anyway? What is the relationship between the tangle of one's feelings and the gesture of compassion? What might it mean to regard the afflicted one as teacher? And one's own afflictions– are they not also teachers? What is the etiquette of one's relationship with these teachers?

These are some of the questions this book asks. And though they are framed in the theater of medicine, each of these questions applies to life wherever it is lived. A hospital or a home where someone is ailing can sometimes turn up the heat, but these dilemmas arise whenever one chooses an authentic life. In matters of soul-making we all begin raw, but each of us can discover a life that remakes us if we do it for real.

·These two words, "craft" and "compassion," then, twine into a single idea: the craft of soul-making in the activity of compassion. The gesture toward a suffering being is at the same time a gesture towards one's own awakening. This craft requires the full gamut of what one is. When one vows to learn compassion, one soon realizes one has pledged one's whole life – from now until one's certain death. We are forever the apprentice with regard to what we don't yet know.

Nothing less than the complete transformation of the self is required.

The way of compassion is radically individual, each of us unique in our virtues and flaws, our passions and our challenges. And as with traveling along any good path, sometimes we meet the craft with poise and grace, sometimes we stumble, blinded by narcissism or a hard heart.

Successes and failures are equally opportunities to refine compassion. Driving home after a hard shift I used to recite my failures of the past twelve hours to myself, but eventually I came to understand "failure" as food for developing self-compassion.

One is immeasurably enriched by diligently walking the path with one's eyes opened. There may be no other way to mature, deep in one's bones. Making soul chamber by chamber, chamber by chamber making soul.

Every day a healthcare provider steps into the hospital or home can be like stepping into a craftsperson's workshop with the grounded enthusiasm of an apprentice of what one doesn't know. Which is to say, every workday is an opportunity to learn.

Step One

Self-Compassion

1

How the Light Gets In

Recently while teaching the craft of compassion in a large drug rehabilitation facility, one worker raised the question of helping addicts heal from shame.

"They are so consumed with self-hate," he said.

He, like almost all sitting in the room, was himself a recovering addict so I asked, "How did you heal from your years of addiction, from your own shame?"

"Well, I let go and let God. I was brought to my knees," he said.

Everyone nodded in assent. I also nodded in assent remembering how I was brought to my knees as a homeless teenage druggie. Unpacking this collective moment of recognition we were able to speak of the nature of genuine self-compassion.

I quoted Leonard Cohen's well-known lyrics: "Forget about your perfect offering. There is a crack in everything. That's how the light gets in."

How do we accept our radiant imperfection? How does humiliation transform into humble acceptance and tenderness for ourselves?

Latin offers the phrase *amor fati*, to "love one's fate." which I would argue describes the foundational stratum of self-love. *One's fate* – not you have chosen but what has been chosen for you. These parents, siblings, ancestors. This body and gender. The delights and terrors of your childhood and the hard-wiring of your character.

What awakens love of one's fate and the sustaining of self-compassion? A spontaneous song of gratitude comes from recognizing that waking or sleeping we forever bask in gift.

Everything, every moment presents as gift – from the vastness of the universe to this very small life to your very next breath.

In the call and response between oneself and the world, one perceives the gift nature of everything and sings "thank you." This simple thank you makes it possible to love one's fate and provides the most reliable source of self-compassion.

It is gratitude that allows one to love the gamut of oneself without judgement, unfettered.

In the years I was recovering from homelessness I kept a "Gratitude Journal" in which I wrote ten things at the end of each day for which I was grateful. My little girl's laughter; the striations of red and magenta in a sunset; the small ways I was learning to be a human being.

As I continued, learning gratitude became a spiritual practice in its own right. As I advanced into the complexities of living an adult life off the street, learning to love my fate became key to broadening and deepening gratitude and self-compassion.

So which came first – the chicken (gratitude) – or the egg (self-compassion)? Well, gratitude does give birth to self-compassion. There is no self-compassion until one can say "thank you" for being alive.

And self-compassion undeniably gives birth to gratitude, truly and profoundly.

Our ideas of causality are confused by the radiant truth of love.

Which came first?

Emphatically both – which makes the love of one's fate vibrant and durable. Whether one enters the door of *gratitude* or *self-compassion* one arrives in the same place.

The authentic interrogation of loving one's fate arises in any circumstance where one is undone by the unforeseen.

For example, you've lost your job. The father of your children has left you for another man. Your grandmother who you thought would live forever has suddenly died. Your doctor has just informed you that you have multiple sclerosis.

I have sometimes asked friends or patients, "what have you learned from your heart condition (or cancer or AIDS or addiction and recovery, etc) that you could not have learned any other way?" A pregnant question to be sure, one that invites the ethos of loving one's fate. When I was diagnosed with multiple sclerosis five years ago, it was my turn to ask that question of myself and ask it fully and completely.

Time to walk my walk.

MS found me a stubbornly young and arrogant man when a range of "symptoms" I'd seen from the outside as a nurse now took *my* body. Falling down in public and unable to get up, incontinent of urine and shit, a unreliable set of legs, sleepless and out of my mind on steroid therapy, losing my eyesight not knowing if it was mine to be blind.

Etc.

Early on, not yet recovered from my first exacerbation, I hiked to my refuge on the Big Sur coast to spend two weeks alone in prayer and reflection. It took eight hours to hike what I knew to be an hour walk and I didn't know if I'd be able to walk out. This was *amor fati* proper.

"Let go and let God." I had to give up the fetish of certainty. For twenty years I'd assumed it would be mine to see my older wife through to the end of her life, but that was suddenly far from certain.

Everything – everything – was far from certain.

To my knees.

To my knees.

Now, these years later, only gratitude remains of my passage through MS. Indeed the medicine of gratitude, of embracing my fate, seems tied up with my healing. It's been two years since my last exacerbation and I don't anticipate another. My neurologist, Dr. Russ Shimizu, was shocked at my recent MRI.

I am free of MS. Few would recognize me as someone with an "incurable" neuromuscular disease.

The transformation of humiliation to humility was, like with so many, a passage through dis-ease. The catalyst of that transformation was gratitude.

The recovering addict at the beginning of the essay was able to walk the twelve steps for real and so recognize his passage through addiction as the situation that reconciled him with himself and God.

When I teach Step One I listen closely to people's stories of what cracked them open.

For one woman it was grieving – in her forties – the murder of her teenage boyfriend over two decades after the event. With another woman, committed to healing women who had been sexually violated, it wasn't until her heart completely broke over her own youthful violation that the fuel of her healing practice shifted from rage to love.

A man told me of how being left by his wife for another also split him open with unbearable rage, but he knew that for the sake of their six year old, despising her would be an act of violence against their kid. Initially, he wrote a long and furious letter to his ex but then had to face how he had also betrayed her – including his own extramarital affairs. He didn't send the letter but did send one speaking of his own betrayals.

"Owning it."

This vein of self-reflection extended from this letter to an improvised spiritual practice, his "mantra," when dealing with any offense from anybody, real or perceived was, "I've done that."

When someone would cut him off in traffic: "I've done that."

A grocery clerk is officious and a little rude: "I've done that."

These three and others showed me how the ordinary and extraordinary wounds between men and women let the light of self-compassion in.

The essential question in all of these stories – and in your story – is, what has cracked you open in this life?

How do you relate to your actual life as a kind friend might?

2

Being Beloved

Self-compassion is making one's life a strong and tender vehicle so that compassion for others can move through. Self-compassion is the eye of the needle through which the thread must pass if you are to meet another with compassion.

Gratitude is the elixir that transforms the sometimes bitter taste of one's fate to nectar, transforms the bereft sense of being abandoned to the recognition of being beloved. When I spoke to addicts of the dreaded, sacred moment of being brought to my knees by illness they understood because the illness of addiction had brought each of them to their knees, each made vulnerable to being systematically altered by surrendering to being beloved.

Being beloved.

The previous chapter spoke of loving one's fate as the substratum and the spiritual practice of gratitude for being alive, the key to *amor fati*. Also key to self-compassion is knowing one is beloved.

John Makransky, in his superb *Awakening Through Love: Unveiling Your Deep Goodness*, writes of spiritually drawing to oneself the "benefactors" – recognizing and visualizing those who have extended love to you since you were a child. "We discover love's transformative and liberating power first by receiving love more fully, then by offering it more inclusively, and finally by becoming a reflex of it from the ground of our being. That is one way to describe the path to enlightenment," writes Makransky. It is basic to Buddhist teaching that the self is made up of non-self elements. This is most certainly true of self-compassion. "Feel free to include your pet as a benefactor. Pets often take such joy in our happiness that it's natural to include them among the benefactors."

Of course one extends the circle of benefactors to those beings that exemplify selfless love – perhaps Christ or the Blessed Virgin, Buddha or Mahatma Gandhi. In this field of benevolence one sits still and accepts that one is beloved.

A simple and profound practice.

Dr. Kristin Neff, professor of Human Development at University of Texas, Austin, has made her life's work researching self-compassion. She writes of three elements of self-compassion: self-kindness, a recognition of common humanity, and mindfulness.

Cynthia's story shows how Neff's elements can play themselves out in the work life of a healthcare provider. She taught me how self-kindness is often about letting go of self-blame and, indeed, the understanding that one is beloved.

She was taking care of Mr. Franklin, a drug addict who had just been rejected as a candidate for a heart transplant because of his history of addiction. "He was forty-five and aware that without a new heart he'd likely die soon," she said. His cardiologist had ordered some blood tests and Cynthia's task was to draw the needed blood. He had a permanent central line running up his arm and into his heart because his veins had collapsed with his addiction and we couldn't maintain an ordinary IV. "This was different from the kind I was familiar with and a bit of blood spilled onto his hospital gown. He lit up with fury."

Cynthia, embarrassed, maintained a persona of competence but felt exposed.

"The truth is my face was flushed and for two hours I was distracted and weak-kneed. It was hard for me to focus on my other patients."

Troubled by what had happened, when she had a break she sat down to pray.

Prayer was an opportunity to be kind to herself, to let go of self-accusation. It was at the same time bringing mindfulness to a confusing welter of feelings.

Mindfulness is an essential theme in this book, pervading both reflections on self-compassion and compassion for others. It is mindfulness that cuts through the postures of egotism that paralyze compassion. Dr. Neff writes:

"Mindfulness is a non-judgmental, receptive mind state in which one observes thoughts and feelings as they are, without trying to suppress or deny them. We cannot ignore our pain and feel compassion for it at the same time. At the same time, mindfulness requires that we not be 'over-identified' with thoughts and feelings, so that we are caught up and swept away by negative reactivity."

"What would it be like to be Mr. Franklin and to have afflicted a likely lethal wound to my own heart?" Cynthia asked herself. Her heart ached physically while she thought this.

It was this physical ache that underscored Dr. Neff's final quality of self-compassion: common humanity. It is the recognition of common humanity that is the fulfillment of self compassion in full transparency to the presence of another.

After praying she went to his room to see how he was doing. He immediately began to apologize.

Mr. Franklin knew that the doctors felt his use of drugs had damaged his heart muscle but he didn't look at his condition clinically.

"I'm just trying to make sense out of things,' he explained. "My anger didn't belong to you. Let me tell you something. I know why my heart is all broke up. I've used heroin a long time, and last year I was shooting up with my oldest boy– twenty one years old! – and he overdosed and died. Truth is, I don't deserve another heart."

Cynthia had planned to apologize to Mr. Franklin about what had happened, but his confession, she said, quieted her and shifted her point of view. During her prayer time she had felt the commonality of a wounded heart with Mr. Franklin. But now his words humbled her and she felt great tenderness towards him and herself.

The mindfulness of prayer softened Cynthia to the recognition of common humanity. Both she and Mr. Franklin had been frightened.

As I came to know Cynthia I learned that for her, self-compassion was of a piece with living a meaningful life.

Recalling who she is as a "civilian" after a hard work week was fully intentional. Walking on the beach with a fellow nurse girlfriend and sharing stories of the week and her committed prayer life are two ways she extends compassion to herself.

"At church the minister preached on 'Even as you have done so to the least of these my brethren you have done so unto me' and I wept, thinking of Mr. Franklin and his son. And when I sang gospel with the choir I wept remembering I'm beloved of God. I mean, that's the bottom line when it comes to self-compassion. I can be so petty with myself, but who am I to argue with the Source of unconditional love?"

Cynthia, as they say, hit the nail on the head. She could love herself because she knew she was beloved.

Compassion without self-compassion relies on a fundamental naïveté about human nature and specifically a blindness to one's own nature. It implies that you imagine yourself inexhaustible, or perhaps as stained and unworthy of compassion. Such ideas cut one off from recognizing one's common humanity with others. It also cuts one off from the wellspring that is the Source of compassion.

3

Regard Yourself with Kindness

A compassionate regard for oneself starts with the insistent self-observation: KNOW THYSELF as inscribed by the ancient Greeks in the temple of Apollo at Delphi.

What is the true story of your life? What is the deep river of your suffering and the broad sky of your happiness? Regard yourself with kindness and sympathy. This is the one who will meet the suffering of another. The Buddha said you could search the world over and not find anyone more deserving of love and compassion than yourself. To ignore this guarantees inevitable burnout.

It does not work to practice compassion at one's own expense.

Compassion for ourselves also means doing the hard work of looking at and accepting our own failings. "If we don't find a way of facing the difficult aspects of our souls, a way of looking honestly at our suffering and its causes in order to develop a meaningful mature compassion for ourselves, then regardless of what we do externally, a sense of emptiness and incompleteness will remain in our hearts," writes Lorne Ladner in his excellent book *The Lost Art of Compassion*.

Ladner advocates a rigorous self-scrutiny but self-scrutiny is not self-accusation. It's about how one splits from the happiness of compassion.

The essence of delusion is to imagine the welfare of self and of others to be in any competition whatsoever. To step out of that false division is to step into the possibility of compassion.

Dr. Mary Jaspers attended a workshop I led on the craft of compassion. The workshop opened with Dr. Neff's exercise on developing self-compassion.

First, I had the participants write something about themselves that made them insecure, "not good enough." "Not-good-enough-ness" struck a profound chord for Mary. I had the group write about the way these feelings felt and then how the emotions settled in the body. Finally I read Neff's third step:

"Now I'd like you to think about an imaginary friend who is unconditionally loving, accepting, kind and compassionate. Imagine that this friend can see all your strengths and all your weaknesses, including the aspect of yourself you have just been thinking about. Reflect upon what this friend feels towards you, and how you are loved and accepted exactly as you are, with all your very human imperfections. This friend recognizes the limits of human nature, and is kind and forgiving towards you. In his/her great wisdom this friend understands your life history and the millions of things that have happened in your life to create you as you are in this moment. The particular inadequacy you face is connected to so many things beyond just you, things you didn't necessarily choose. Your genes, your family history, how you were raised, events happening in your life – many things that were outside of your control."

Finally, as per Dr. Neff, I had Mary write herself a letter from this friend.

In medical school. Mary was told that well over 50% of doctors and nurses are adult children of alcoholics. Mary was raised in an alcoholic and drug using family and her feelings of being a small and insufficient child were with her throughout her medical training and in her practice as an MD.

"I so much wanted to save them but there was nothing I could do! I was such a good girl." she said with a bitter laugh. As a child of an alcoholic myself I certainly knew what it was to carry this belief in my insufficiency into my adulthood.

How very common this is for we who commit to helping others.

It was the voice of Mother Earth that addressed the doctor who yesterday was a little girl.

Dear Mary,

You are enough.

You are kind enough. You are generous enough. Strong enough; smart enough; good enough.

DOING ENOUGH!

You are working on becoming careful. You are working on becoming thoughtful. To have work to do is part of the Divine Plan. Go to that work with an open heart.

Remember your small child – she was always enough. Remember to tell her.

When you are feeling "not enough" STOP. Sit in the awareness that every being is perfect.

Breathe deep and release that tension of unreasonable demand. Rest in the expanse of the peace of All That Is and rejoin the love of All Your Relations.

Now go forth with that knowledge.

Love,

Your Mother

Step Two

Compassion for Another

4

Thresholds

Threshold. Boundary. Me and you, or more formally, "I and Thou." Each of us wrapped in our skin, our fate, but – "meeting" nonetheless.

Self-compassion is the eye of spiritual attentiveness through which we must pass if we are to learn what it is to *live* compassion. The passage is direct, cut from necessity and clarity. In loving oneself one is available to love another. One meets oneself in the love of someone else.

"The individual is not just a separate being, but by his very existence presupposes a collective relationship," writes C. G. Jung.

No man or woman is an island. And even islands are not truly islands. They do not float on the surface of the sea and drift hither and thither. Islands rise up from common submerged ground. Whether the common ground of humans is seen or not, it is nonetheless the ground we walk on from conception to death. Our commonality is the ground of compassion.

"Know thyself" is critical in the awakening of self-compassion but it is also a call to the knowledge of shared humanity. As Glaser puts it, "At bottom, we are left with the incontrovertible truth that every being, friend, foe or stranger wishes for happiness and wishes to be free of suffering, just as we do."

Our patients present a vivid mirror and our measure of mercy is continuous with the mercy we extend to the one revealed by them. It's the mirroring aspect I want to emphasize here. The mirror that is another face is the continuity between one's intimate self and a suffering other that calls for compassion.

The passage across the threshold is archetypal before it is personal. One centers and empties out so the space is clear of projection and you can receive another – I to Thou.

Explicitly and implicitly, I and Thou is a major theme in this book. Myself and everyone I interviewed spoke of the circumstance of a genuine *meeting* being precisely the moment of compassion. All speak of what the French call *disponibilité,* a spiritual availability to the person of the other. For Rabbi Carla Howard and Catholic Katherine Brown-Saltzman, "emptying" serves this availability.

"All real life is meeting," wrote Martin Buber, and all real meeting, I to Thou, calls on the spirit of kindness by virtue of being a *real* meeting. Hasidic Jews say an angel is born whenever two truly meet in this basic reciprocity. Christ said, "Whenever two or more of you are gathered in my name, there am I among you."

The threshold we cross to the understanding of the common humanity is the true nature of the village. It is the very ground of compassion.

The threshold is what makes a village. It is what makes compassion possible in any given soul, in any village, including a hospital.

The threshold is the border that separates and connects everyone in the village. In a hospital it runs through every interaction between staff and patients, patients and their families, patients and one another. As a community presence the threshold is pervasive and invisible: invisible because it's pervasive and also because it's so often ignored.

Above all, the threshold is where two stories connect. We meet another always at the threshold –of our own world, of our stories, of a village. All of us carry stories from which we construct a compassionate life. Stories of friends, kin, our own struggles, stories of patients we've taken care of. This is the wealth we bring to the edge between ourselves and the community of patients and their families. These stories are spiritual food that nourishes something deathless, something eternal.

5

Compassion Is an Action

There can be a confusion between "feeling" compassion and the life that is actually living compassion. Yet feeling is intimately involved with realizing and living compassion.

Sympathy for someone's joy and sorrow leads feeling beyond the edge of self to meet an other. Feeling is the current between you and I. In this way, feeling is not "precious," self-involved or self-important.

Instead it is responsive. Compassion is the intelligence of a feeling heart.

However, it is those that frighten us or for whom we feel no familiarity, no easy warmth, who call us to the deeper truths of compassion.

Compassion is an intent and an expression – an action – that comes from somewhere deeper and broader than feeling. Nowhere is this fact demonstrated more clearly than in the life of St. Francis of Assisi. It was a leper that opened the path of compassion for the young man who was to become St. Francis. Francis was sincere in his love of God and his desire to serve the poor. However, he could not bear the sight of the lepers, and he could see that because of this, his otherwise committed life had a hollowness to it, a refusal to fully live by what he knew to be true.

He cried in prayer that he might be relieved of the repulsion he felt in the presence of lepers. The despair that such a prayer might go unanswered left him raw. It was in the stupor of that despair that he met a leper on the road and wept. He recognized him as Christ and embraced him.

Every healthcare worker knows, like Francis, what it is to shrink in disgust.

Martha was frightened of Robert at first. She was very aware of the "monster" on the floor long before she became his nurse. Doctors were rushing in and out of his room because the sight of him unnerved them; nurses whispering about his tragedy. Some nurses refused to take care of him at all.

Thirty-nine years old, with AIDS and a rare form of skin cancer, his body was a mass of scabs and smelly necrotic tissue. Martha first spied him as a furtive voyeur. One of her patients shared a room with him, and she caught a quick glance of him and his wife through a crack in the drawn curtain. She prayed like hell she'd never be his nurse.

In the divine scheme of things, Martha told me later, prayers to protect a closed heart are apparently not highly regarded. The next day Robert was her patient.

She paused before his door and said, "Show me how. I am so limited and confused. Please show me how." Perhaps this prayer is highly regarded by whomever hears prayers. When she walked in, she was quickly shown the possibility, indeed the reality, of Robert's beauty.

His teenaged daughter, Lucy, the same age as Martha's daughter, Lydia, was at the bedside lovingly tending to her dad. Martha caught his reflection also in the eyes of his wife, LaRhonda, before she looked fully at him.

It was a moment for Martha very much like Francis's meeting with the leper.

"It completely changed my life and definitely changed my nursing," she told me. "I was able to see him from a totally new perspective when I saw how LaRhonda and Lucy saw him. Ever since that moment, when I have a negative reaction to a patient, I *know* it's about me and I try to look at the patient through the eyes of love.

"This is a well-loved man, " Martha said to LaRhonda.

"Oh yes," said LaRhonda. "We just give back the love he's given us."

Martha had stumbled into a story of relationships. She could no longer see a monster. There was a radiance in the room. Nothing less than that.

Robert was full of light.

His cancer went from bad to worse. One night Martha walked in and found that, in his agitation, he'd torn off a portion of his nose. The clotting factor of his blood was low, as it sometimes is with certain cancers. He was literally in a pool of blood and choking on it.

She tried all she knew. "I thought ice would tighten the blood vessels since pressure wasn't working. After a half-hour the bleeding finally stopped. With reluctance I tied his hands and feet and gave him a shot of sedative. He could kill himself by tearing at his body!"

At 3 a.m. it was her break time and she decided to spend it in Robert's room praying.

"He had so frightened me before I saw his beauty. I felt I had something important to learn by praying alongside him."

His appearance hadn't changed in the least, but there was that uncanny light upon it.

"When he stirred and opened his eyes I walked over to him and said, 'You can let go, Robert. You needn't cling to this life. When you feel it's time to let go, you can trust it.'"

Alert, mute, calm – he listened.

When she returned to work a few days later, the doctor had written a dying patient protocol directive: hang a morphine drip, increase it as necessary to patient's comfort, don't be concerned about changes in vital signs.

After watching Robert disintegrate for weeks, a morphine drip seemed merciful. And when LaRhonda asked Martha to turn up the morphine, she did so, not knowing whether she was inviting the death of a man whose beauty she had come to see.

"It's time for him to move on," said LaRhonda.

After midnight just as Martha entered the room Robert took one long gasp.

It was in fact his last breath.

"Go well, Robert," Martha prayed, while Lucy wailed, "Daddy, Daddy, Daddy." Later when Lucy took out a camera to photograph her father's spent self, Martha realized again that for his daughter, Robert was never anything less than beautiful.

The love of Robert's family directed Martha to the soul behind the leper's mask, and so she was able to meet that soul first and foremost. It was much harder, I think, for me to find Norbert's soul than it was for Martha to find Robert's.

Norbert was a handsome sixty-five-year-old man with advanced-stage pancreatic cancer. Deadly. And he knew it. While admitting him, I asked him about his life, where he was from, his career and such.

Norbert, it turns out, was from the East Coast and as a young man had been a graduate student whiz-kid in biology. In the early forties he was recruited to New Mexico to help with the war effort. Specifically Los Alamos – the development of the first atomic bomb.

"Really?" I said. "I wrote a book that had three chapters on the Manhattan Project." I was taken in the moment by Norbert's easy charm, and my years of studying these things made for a pleasure in hearing the inside gossip on Oppenheimer, Teller, Szilard, and the rest. I was startled awake when he said, "In '44, I made a fuss. 'What am I doing here? I'm a biologist, not a physicist!' And so they transferred me to Tennessee, and I spent the rest of my career on biological weapons."

When I left his room, I became aware of the impact of his last disclosure. I was thoroughly split between the surface conversation on one hand and my deep judgment on the other. The banality of evil was revealed as a pleasant man who had given his life over to perfecting the means of mass murder.

I took care of my other patients distractedly. Of course I vetoed calling him to task on the moral substance of his life. It was strangely tempting, yet obviously utterly childish, and under the circumstances, would have been entirely cruel. Nonetheless, my mind kept rehearsing all the passion and eloquence that I would never speak.

I did not want to take care of Norbert that night or any other night. I did not want anyone to take care of Norbert. I didn't care if he lived or died. A couple of hours later while I was still steaming in these thoughts his call light went off.

Coming into his room, I found him panicked, soaked in sweat, gripping at his side in excruciating pain. I turned on my heel to get some morphine, and when I returned I took a couple of long breaths as I injected it in his IV line. Then I grabbed a cool washrag to sponge his sweaty brow.

"I've been waking up this way lately. I get so frightened and confused. I don't want to die." I sat with him for half an hour, breathing with him until the panic settled and the morphine took him back to sleep.

It is a common mistake to believe compassion is about "feeling" compassionate. Feeling compassion can be a sweet thing, but sometimes one feels compassionate and sometimes one doesn't. In truth, compassion is about stepping forth regardless of your feelings or judgments simply because that is what you are called to do.

Sure, I'd rather Norbert had lived a decent life slinging tofu burgers, the better to die a peaceful death. However, his panic reminded me of the irrelevance of my opinions. In such moments the greater truth is about getting myself - my opinions, prejudgments, even morals - out of the way so the spirit of kindness can do its thing.

I don't know if I "felt" compassion for Norbert, or even warmth. I do know it was mine that night to sit beside a man who'd awakened stripped to all but cold fear in the darkness that would soon swallow his life.

6

Joy of Your Joy, Sorrow of Your Sorrow

The Buddha defines compassion with such clarity. Compassion, he says, is sympathetic joy and sympathetic sorrow – sorrow over another's sorrow and delight over another's delight.

This is the stuff of profound teaching. It is sacred for its homely truth, rhymes well with "Do unto others as you would have them do unto you."

These ancient understandings can seem abstract but when we *live by them* they are vivid, warm, sometimes intimate.

"How far you go in this life," writes George Washington Carver, "depends on you being tender with the young, compassionate with the aged, sympathetic with the striving, and tolerant of the weak and the strong, because one day you will have been all of these."

Sympathy is grounded in the fact that we, or someone we love, did or will experience the same thing as those we take care of. It's just a matter of time before you or a loved one is ill, perhaps hospitalized. One out of two men and one in three women will die of cancer. We know, don't we, it's just a matter of time before you or someone you dearly loves dies.

We diminish our own hearts if we deny the jeopardy that is the common truth of being human and mortal.

Sorrow and joy are the fabric of the everyday, renewed with each new life experience.

William Blake writes: "Joy and woe are woven fine / A clothing for the soul Divine."

Sorrow and joy are the raw material out of which a compassionate life is discovered and lived.

If we live our lives consciously – that is to say with the intent of extending compassion to ourselves and all that we meet – then all that we are and all that we do is the act of weaving.

This weaving is an act of joy as is opening to another's sorrow. Meeting sorrow we are freed from our self-preoccupation, which is where our suffering renews itself.

Compassion is, in fact, joy.

We hold our experiences of sorrow and joy as stories and these stories instruct our souls in the range of experience that makes every human life a common and blessed thing.

The work of a healthcare provider who seeks to awaken compassion involves gathering his or her own stories like seeds. They hold the possibility of sprouting and, in time perhaps, bear fruit for nourishment or flowers for beauty.

We all know sympathetic joy.

Your friend's HIV test comes back clean; your sister had her first child and she's a doll; the lump in your aunt's breast turns out to be benign; your cousin finally got out of a very bad marriage and she's starting to smile again.

I emphasize suffering not to deny the sheer blessed fact of being alive but because we would rather deny suffering. But the denial of suffering is a machine that itself generates such suffering!

Joy that relies on the denial of suffering is a superficial and fragile fiction. Eventually it will be undone. Misery can be hidden away in the shadow of an overly optimistic culture, but when it is brought out into the open as the common ground of suffering, it can awaken compassion.

In this sense, linking your personal suffering to that of your patients becomes a gift to you and through you, a gift to them.

A few examples:

Roland has AIDS, and will likely die soon. He's only thirty-five. I lost my friend Charlie, a Vietnam vet who worked with the criminally insane, to AIDS when he was the same age. My friend Alberto had AIDS too. A month before Alberto died I did a Tarot reading for him and of course he picked up the Death card. He was so relieved to talk about it openly. All of his friends in his large gay community had lost loved ones and it was unbearable to them that it was Alberto's turn. "It's time," he said.

My youngest brother, Paul, was psychotic. Mad, he wandered off into the New Mexico mountains and died there. Every young psychotic patient could be my brother.

Carl is homeless, in his early thirties, an addict and diabetic, cellulitis oozing on his left foot, soon to be an amputee. What broke him so? I was homeless for three years as a teenager. I'll know how to love him remembering how fierce and cold it can get.

Each of these stories of my friends and loved ones is intimately real to me, but when linked to another's suffering it is no longer mine. They are now not a burden but an opportunity for connection, which offers a kind of freedom. A naïve individualism infects the western world, so much so that we imagine freedom to be a lonely, even alienated thing. The kind of freedom I speak of here is not independence but interdependence, the vibrant community of we who sustain one another and sometimes set one another free beyond the edge of our own precious but small life.

Clutching at personal suffering amplifies and distorts it.

Sympathetic joy and sorrow delivers us into a lived understanding of being of the human community. Sorrow is one eye and joy is the other. With the two together we can see any situation with depth.

Our patients are ourselves. Grandmother and grandfather, mother, father. brother, sister. Friend, neighbor or the strangest of strangers. They deliver us to the family and community within us, to the community and next of kin that we are.

Our patients present an opportunity for self-compassion because we are not different from them.

We walk through the life that we've lived even as we walk through whatever comes our way, the two meeting each other in a field of sympathetic sorrow and joy. Here we can see sorrow and joy as the possibility of compassion that lives within the stories of our lives and the lives we bear witness to.

The spirit of kindness is deathless. Perhaps you've met it in moments but it existed long before your birth and will persist long after you're gone. It is the bedrock from which we all spring, the God that is love and the love that is God.

I call the place of shared humanity the village. You are – we are all - of the village simply by virtue of being born.

Those who can meet another's joy with joy, those who have transformed a portion of their suffering into compassion are walking a very old path.

Many have walked this way.

6

I-It and I-Thou

A hospital, any hospital, has a wild streak to it, a rawness, sometimes a heartlessness. Most employees know the impact of this aspect of institutionalized medicine, the weariness from sleeplessness, the steady diet of carbohydrates and coffee, the burnout that sometimes seems endemic.

Of course healthcare providers know the bitterness of this heartlessness but it is the patients who know it in full. By my estimation Martin Buber is the thinker that writes most clearly of what it is that entraps us, and what frees us.

Buber wrote of I-Thou and I-It relationships. I-Thou describes authentic, reciprocal relationships. The language of common humanity: "I recognize you and you recognize me. We know ourselves to be other and present to one another."

I-It often describes relationships in a modern hospital. There is no true relationship, and the patient can be just a mass of tasks to be done. Or a nonentity dangling invisibly from a diagnosis.

Sometimes this is explicit. "The MI (myocardial infarction) in 568." "The COPD-er (congestive obstructive pulmonary disease) in 411". While suffering is excruciatingly present, the person who suffers often goes unseen or is marginalized in the rush of moving from one task to another.

Mr. Charles, I was told at change of shift, was bipolar (and we know how *they* are . . .) with a history of addiction. Noncompliant. As a black, homeless Vietnam vet, he knew what it was to be a non-person, a "no-thing." An It. The haze of labels with which the doctors and nurses communicated about his care obliterated him altogether. He was no longer a man with a story.

To be someone with a story is to be a Thou. Without a story, one is an It.

I told Mr. Charles that I'd recently traveled to Vietnam with Dr. Ed Tick and a handful of American veterans for peacemaking and healing.

"Why would vets return to Vietnam if they weren't going to kill gooks?" he asked. He used the word American soldiers used to strip the Vietnamese enemy of their stories.

I told him we broke bread with Viet Cong vets in the Mekong delta and NVA vets in Hanoi.

"Damn!" was his incredulous response, "I ain't ever going back to that hellhole."

The enemy in any given war is always an It and an essential part of the training of a soldier is to convince them that the enemy is not human in the same way *we* are. My friend Marty who accompanied me to Vietnam tells me of going through a wallet of a recently killed Vietnamese and looking at a photograph of his wife and kids.

·No longer a gook.

Post Traumatic Stress Disorder shows us the profound wound of killing and *gookifying* the enemy. It shows the soul's ineffective attempt to protect itself from this wound.

Likewise, we can commit atrocities on the bodies and minds of patients as long as they're "Its". All professions have their shadows. Maybe this is a soul's perverse effort at self-protection when the suffering one bears witness to in an ordinary work day is incomprehensible.

Never a soldier, I learned the logic of I-It in nursing school and have seen medical students learning its ways in teaching hospitals.

As institutions, hospitals have a thousand and one ways of depriving patients of their humanity. My second semester in nursing school I was nothing if not innocent when I began clinical rotations in a small community hospital. I was assigned an elderly woman patient who knew she was dying and refused all extraordinary measures to keep her alive. Her lung sounds were greatly congested, so my assignment was to extend a suction catheter in her mouth, an un-traumatizing way of removing secretions. She clenched her teeth. I then, feeling a little nauseous, began pushing a new suction catheter up her nose. She looked at me with an expression of pure hatred. I thought: "You are absolutely right. This is contemptible."

When I told my nursing instructor that I couldn't follow through with this, she said, "You must. You cannot refuse a patient a measure of comfort."

Later in the hall a fellow student found me weeping. "I think I'm going to hell for what we do here," I said.

Sandra, a good Christian woman, reassured me, but I wasn't being at all literal. When an act of cruelty is described as a comfort measure, hell is not far away.

The pressure of tasks encourages depersonalization. In the cascade of doing this-and-that, and the push-and-pull of needs and sometimes emergencies, a healthcare provider quickly develops an incentive for damage control, and with it comes a tightening of the heart.

"What is the minimum I can give this patient so I can go on to the next one, and the one after that?"

It's entirely possible to hang an IV, give pills, take vital signs, and scarcely notice the patient. A longer task during which a healthcare provider might actually meet the patient – an admission from ER, an elaborate dressing change – is often met with irritation because there is so much to do.

Of course, the pressure is greatly amplified by poor staffing. The suffering of the patients becomes "my" ordeal. "How in God's name will I make it through this shift?" We are susceptible to an institutionalized narcissism, in which the afflictions of the profession loom larger than those of the patients.

This essential, institutional double bind cuts both ways: "I'm here to take care of you – but please don't ask anything of me because you can't even imagine how busy I am." The patient becomes an It, but so does the healthcare worker. It divides healthcare workers from their hearts and generates burnout.

There is an internal I-It split within themselves.

It is the essence of – in fact describes – alienation when one is relating to others as It.

When one is doing so, one is no longer an "I."

For an employee, a hospital can become a prison in which one lives a life that is not one's own. One endures this life and yearns for the life that won't be lived until re-careering or retirement.

I remembered Marianna from the years we had worked alongside each other, especially her repeated self-accusations that she ever decided to be a nurse. "I was so young when I made that choice, but in five years I'll be retired!"

Marianna was forcibly "retired" with brain cancer and was my patient one long night. She held a mirror to all on oncology. She was largely nonverbal when I took care of her but when she spoke it was incomprehensible. Expressive aphasia. Her neurological situation sabotaged her capacity to complain.

A fierce fate: years of complaining about patient's complaints and about having chosen a profession that she'd be lost in a sea of complaint, and now? Drowning in inexpressible complaint as a patient.

I have learned that it is possible – even necessary – to walk the tightrope between the I-It of nursing's endless tasks and the I-Thou of meeting the patient. The soul of the healthcare worker is at stake, as are the meaning and joy that are possible in the healing professions.

For years I'd come home after three twelve-hour night shifts to my wife, who had spent those days practicing as a therapist and a teacher. We'd go into the long "debriefing" – always as storytelling. This was absolutely necessary to find our way back to each other – and my way back to "civilian" life. One doesn't speak of the details of the work in polite company.

Pre-op enemas at a cocktail party?

And then there's one's child. I came home after a dear patient died, slept for a few hours, and picked up my daughter, Nicole, from elementary school. I was bleary-eyed as we watched *Sesame Street*.

Mr. Hooper had just died, and Maria was explaining to Big Bird that he was never coming back. I burst into tears. Nicole asked me if I was crying about my father. "Yes, and my patient Marianna also."

I could see that Nicole understood what it is to think with her heart.

7

Letting the World Change You

Conversation with Heather Watkins, RN

Heather Watkins is a nurse who sees the profession of nursing as a way of spiritual transformation. Specifically, she has been transformed by caring for the dying both as an oncology nurse and in hospice care. I've worked alongside Heather and been struck by her quiet, warm manner at the bedside of the ill, her perceptiveness, and her willingness to let her heart break in heartbreaking circumstances and thus be changed by the work of compassion.

Heather's story about caring for an American Nazi's death is not naïve nor, God forbid, pro-Nazi. She moves from a simple profound premise: we don't always choose who we are called to care for. The transformation for the patient and Heather underscores that it's not ours to choose who is worthy of compassion.

Michael: What is compassion?

Heather: In the movie *The Motorcycle Diaries* one of the characters said, "Let the world change you and you can change the world." I think in many ways this describes compassion. When you are willing to step into an open heart and mind, you are changed and you are an agent of change for those around you.

Michael: I befriended you as an oncology nurse and now you work hospice. Throughout your career, death and dying has been the field where you let the world change you.

Heather: I used to work in an oncology unit in Austin, Texas. Everyone had "do not resuscitate" orders. There was a realistic attitude about these patient's terminal states that made for an openness, a certain amount of self-reflection, a deep heart connection with them. It drew me out. Dying chips away illusion and delusion. It drew me into an alliance with the patients, which changed me as well as them because of the real work that could be done.

I went from there to another hospital in Simi Valley, California – a very different scene. Huge bedsores that you could slide a fist into. Patients with no quality of life kept alive by dialysis. It was hard to meet the challenges of people who were in this world only because of medical technology.

When I got a job at a large and prestigious hospital I took it to be the high point of my career. I worked on the oncology and bone marrow transplant floor, where people look for miracles. And we tried to offer miracles. Unfortunately, in the process some realities were missed.

I had a seventeen-year-old patient with recurrent leukemia who had developed graft-versus-host disease of the gut. That meant he was bleeding and nothing could be done. He was bloated from head to toe and was being transfused with blood on a daily basis. He barely had the strength to speak, but was able to say that all he wanted was to go home. He was in a room by himself on an air mattress. That was his life.

What was heartbreaking as a nurse was that there was no conversation with the family about the fact that he was not going to survive. He was going to die, and he just wanted to go home, but nobody was being straight. Nobody.

In my opinion, closure at the end of a life is spiritually necessary to help the soul move on. I did my best to sit with that boy, just sit with him, hold his hand, and let him know that he was heard. It was the only gesture I could give him. I didn't feel empowered enough at that hospital, and, in all honesty, I was too young to know how to do it well.

At another hospital in Los Angeles, I had two terminal patients with AIDS, but the doctors weren't telling the families. I was more secure as a nurse so I spoke directly with those families. I said, "You know he's terminal." Both responded, "That's what we thought, but nobody has talked to us about it."

I think medical staff is afraid that if we're open with families and patients there will be an explosion of grief or anger, but I've never seen that happen, not even once. The response has always been, "Oh that's what we thought," and they were so relieved that somebody was willing to have that conversation with them. For the patients, then they could make real decisions about their own treatment. They'd look at the IV fluids and nutrition running into their veins and say, "Well I guess this is kind of pointless."

Michael: Tell me about hospice.

Heather: Like in the hospital, the question remains: Do we really see our patients? The best example I can give is a German-American Nazi man I took care of. He was in his fifties, in and out of jail, swastikas tattooed all over his body. Before I came to work with him, he removed his guns from the back of his front door.

Bringing his case to my hospice team was quite a challenge. There was, of course, much resistance to the Nazi element. I wasn't afraid. I think compassion requires a certain fearlessness. If you're afraid, you erect defenses and they prevent you from really seeing the person before you. You expect you will be harmed, and that feeds the harm that's already there. With compassion or any kind of healing work you have to take the risk that you may get hurt.

I saw a man who had been hurt and was almost begging for someone to see beyond his defenses. He was struggling to know how to be seen. He had so much fear he didn't know how to invite anyone in.

In the course of my first visit I listened to him without judgment. My acknowledging his experiences as he saw them allowed the door to open for me. When I'd take his blood pressure and his heart rate I could see he was at ease.

Gradually he began to trust me. He began to trust my ability to run things effectively, which was important to him. And because I was willing to listen to him he essentially did what a Catholic might call a confession right near the end of his life. He talked about what he would have done differently, how he lacked patience and the capacity to express love openly. He asked me how to be in the world in a better way.

He had hired a caregiver named Teresa, a Native American woman. One time he wanted her to do something and barked out an order as usual, but then he corrected himself and asked in a kind way. Then he looked at me and said, "Was that okay?"

By the end of his life he reconciled with his mother with whom he had a volatile relationship. She took care of him his final two weeks. I remember him opening his eyes and calling his mother, "Come here." When she came, he kissed her on the forehead and said, "I love you."

I believe this would not have happened if someone hadn't been willing to put aside the stereotypes and fears and be willing to listen to him and be changed. My staff still speaks of it. We were successful in helping him close his life in a positive way and go on more evolved. That's all we can hope for.

As nurses, as people, it seems to be about loving the person before you, regardless of who they are and listening to their stories without judgment. This is where healing begins.

8

Hasten Slowly

Walking the tightrope of institutional nursing is about crafting time. In professional training they call it "time management," but getting all your work done in the allotted twelve hours is the least of it – that is, if you take compassion seriously. Crafting time requires learning to shift from the merciless rush of task work to dropping into an open ease at the bedside of the patient.

During the Renaissance they'd say, "Hasten slowly." In nursing it's "Hasten when you must, but when you're called to the bed of suffering, stop." Without stopping, without hesitating at the door to breathe, there is no room for the spirit of kindness to arrive. You have chased it away, and the patient knows this immediately.

It takes years to learn this. The hospital is a place of training in this most peculiar craft. My first efforts were none too impressive. I lasted four months before I was fired.

Hell hath no fury like an understaffed nurse. I had twelve patients that particular night, three times as much as any well-staffed hospital would allow. No nurse's aide. Neuro floor. High demand for acuity. A sea of sputum and desperation.

I'd rushed in and out of Mrs. Green's room twice in the shift. Assessment. Vital signs. Meds. Fifty-five years old, yellow, lung sounds liquid, belly hugely distended. End-stage cirrhosis. Pickled her liver with alcohol.

At 4 a.m. she called me to her room. "Am I dying?"

I paused, stumbled for words. Is a euphemism asked for? Does one answer such naked directness with euphemism? "Your condition is grave," I responded.

While I tended to my other patients, Mrs. Green called her husband at home, and he came to her bedside. I walked into her room to take her morning vital signs the very moment she died tenderly in her husband's arms.

Her last breath was the proverbial straw that broke the camel's back. I knew I was obligated to begin CPR, send her husband into the hall, and call a code blue – the big guns – to resuscitate her. That would buy her perhaps three days in an intensive care unit being tortured. I was, of course, moving on automatic: enraged and putting my foot down.

Not skillful.

I wanted no part in the routinized institutional cruelty of it all. I walked to the charge nurse and said, "Mrs. Green just died."

"Call a code."

"I won't."

"You must."

The charge nurse herself called the code team in. Her husband stood in the hallway weeping while a guard was at the doorway between him and the room. I paged the doctor frantically to get an order to call off the code as her husband requested. Not getting an answer I stepped into her room. After watching the code team deliver another round of electroshocking her heart I announced, "This is obscene. Her husband wants this to stop. Let the woman go."

Twenty minutes later, cardiac monitor flat line, Mrs. Green lay in the disarray of a woman raped on her deathbed. The code team wandered off, and while I closed her eyes, speaking to her, speaking to her husband, I said, "I am so sorry." I removed her IV line and tidied her up so he could be alone with her.

I was fired the next day.

There are thresholds and the violation of thresholds. Crossing over at the moment of death is the ultimate crossing of threshold. "What would Jesus do?" I asked the nun who fired me.

She was silent to my inquiry.

Had I known about hastening slowly, I'd never had made a beautiful death such high drama. I'd have paused before the holy moment I'd stumbled onto. I would have stopped and allowed my awareness to recollect itself and then have asked her husband if he wanted me to initiate resuscitating her. If he'd said "yes," I would have done so. And if "no," I would have left him with her for an hour to say his good-byes. Then I would tell the charge nurse that Mr. Green says his wife died an hour ago. No one would try to revive a cold corpse. Cunning for sure and our retrospective selves are impressive in their wisdom and good sense, but I could have stopped an act of violence from happening if I hadn't panicked before such a simple death.

Or so I thought. When I shared my strategy with my friend Dr. Leslie Blackhall, she laughed. "I once taught an in-service with physicians and asked who had performed a code on patients after rigor mortis had set in. Virtually all of them raised their hands. 'Why?' I asked. 'There was no do not resuscitate order,' I was told. 'Did you really imagine you could raise the dead?' I laughed in response."

As a doctor concerned with the care of the dying she knows how grossly overused code blue is. "Coding was devised for cardiac arrest, but now it's used as obligatory, as if a necessity. The effect is that we prolong the process of dying in ways that often means torturing the patient until they give up the ghost."

The place of threshold is not a place of rules. The concepts of threshold and boundary offer a scaffolding for the compassionate imperative but every situation must be met on its own merits. For Mrs. Green, code blue was a gross violation. But I was to emphatically find out that is not always the case.

The threshold is a place for interpreting what's appropriate in every moment, with every meeting.

Mr. Pedrozo was a Filipino patient, sixty-five and very, very ill. End stage renal disease. His daughters, Clara and Lourdes, attended him at his bedside.

When his nurse, Toni, met him he was going down. Fast. Because his kidneys were shut down, his lungs were pools of fluid. Multiple systems failure. She arranged for him to have an emergency dialysis to draw off his fluid overload before he drowned.

"Mr. Pedrozo was so much on the edge," she said. "Was there a way to stop his death from being prolonged as hospitals are given to doing?" I thought. At the same time I knew that I'd follow through resuscitation procedures if it came to that. I wasn't sure this was ethical but if I had to I guess I would.

It was from within this turmoil that Toni approached the daughters about a "do not resuscitate" order. They listened respectfully and left the hospital saying they'd talk to their family.

A couple of hours later their brother Reynaldo called, furious. "What, you just want to let my dad go, is that it? That's not what *we* want. His brother is flying in from the Philippines. He hasn't seen him in twenty years. He wants to say good-bye before he goes. Who do you think you are, trying to convince my sisters that we should just let him go?"

Who indeed? Toni was not thinking like a villager, much less a villager from Luzon. "I was thinking like a shell-shocked nurse," she said. In the village, death is not the will of the body pitted against the technology that would try to revive it. "This man was an elder, for God's sake," she said, "and his brother was also an elder and was flying across the ocean to say farewell."

Mr. Pedrozo survived the shift but "coded" on the next shift. Hospital language is so odd sometimes. "Coded" does not mean death, though it could carry death within its possible meanings. A lot of coded patients cannot be revived. Mr. Pedrozo was not one of those. For him, "coded" meant that he had another four days in ICU, largely unconscious. His brother arrived, the two of them met after two decades, and the next day he was coded, again and could not be revived.

These two stories open up a spaciousness, an openness because together they undo the constrictions of dogma, the delusions of certainty.

The activity of compassion sometimes requires "not knowing."

9

Honoring Thresholds

Conversation with Rabbi Carla Howard

Rabbi Howard is a woman of remarkable intelligence, heart, and reflection, for whom crossing thresholds is a spiritual practice. She crosses the threshold to the presence of the ill and dying and gathers to herself awareness and a sense of the sacred nature of compassionate activity. While profoundly informed by the way of the ancestors, Carla listens to the story beneath the story of people who are facing the raw truth of their life. Her insights into the activity of compassion are similar to others I talked to, but here with a Jewish inflection.

"Love your neighbor as yourself," is the sacred intent one carries across the threshold to the bed of the ill.

Carla works with the dying and is the founder of Jewish Hospice Project of Los Angeles.

Michael: Tell me about how you came to care for the dying.

Carla: I am a conservative rabbi with a long history of the study of contemplative Judaism, a student of Rabbi Jonathan Omer-man. I was the Associate Rabbi of the Metivta Center for Contemplative Judaism with Jonathan. Through the study of kabbalah, I came back to join an earlier piece of my life.

I'd been a pre-med student and had worked both in women's healthcare in the early seventies, which was a burgeoning time of women's self help, and also as a journeywoman midwife with the home birth movement at that time.

This was my introduction to pastoral care, long before I became a rabbi. My rabbinate both in rabbinical school and post rabbinical school had to do with pastoral care. Spiritual direction, helping people find a sense of peace. Many Jews fled Judaism to other traditions because Judaism didn't make its meditation tradition very accessible, put it behind locked doors of scholarship and the Hebrew language.

At Metivta, I was the head of the healing center and people started to call me about hospice patients. I wondered why there was no spiritual care for Jewish dying here in Los Angeles, the second largest Jewish city in the world. So we started the Jewish Hospice Project Los Angeles, which offers spiritual care for the dying and their families. We've seen five hundred patients in these years. We don't charge anybody.

We reach out to people in whatever phase of illness they are in. The sooner ill people come to a language of spirituality the more prepared they are for what might evolve. If they come to a language of spirituality when they are diagnosed they are on better ground as opposed to rushing in to define the terms at a late point or at the very end.

Michael: What is the movement of your contemplative practice to the bedside of the ill? How meditation inform your work?

Carla: Judaism has a concept of *kavanah*, meaning the "intentionality" that precedes any ritual act. *Kavanah* is the moment before you take the action to rest and focus the lens and connect with the Source so the action is aligned. This is the way of the ritual act but also any gesture of compassion.

Michael: So as you approach the bedside of the ill you pull back to focus, to connect with *kavanah,* so you meet the sacred reality of what is there?

Carla: That's exactly it. I see most people in their homes. I call on *kavanah* at their doorway before going in. Adonai is the name we address God in our prayers. In Hebrew the doorway, the threshold, has the same root as the name of God. That passageway is where we do a kind of centering, emptying.

Michael: This is also my modus operandi. One acknowledges that one is passing the threshold.

Carla: The *mezuzah* marks the door for that. (A *mezuzah* is a little box with the Jewish declaration of faith written in Hebrew and affixed to the doorjamb.) There is a clearing and you come to meet the face of the Divine with the person in the bed. And the hovering presence over the bed where our tradition tells us the Divine lingers. Our laws tell us that you don't sit at the head of the bed, you sit at the foot. This is from the Talmud.

The line in the Torah, the rubric under which all these behaviors are refined in the different layers of interpretation in Mishnah and Talmud, is "You shall love your neighbor as you love yourself." That is what sets the *kavanah* toward who is in the bed. That is the sacred intent.

Michael: So you are meeting yourself, so to speak. There is a radical peership. You meet the Divine by meeting the other as yourself.

Carla: Yes, that's it.

Michael: There was a "threshold" in your own life that you crossed when you began to look for the Divine in the face of the ill, the dying. What was the moment when you saw that the sacred work that your soul was called to was to serve the Divine at the bedside of the ill?

Carla: There is a chapter in between pre-med and being a rabbi. It involved listening to people's life stories. I was a documentary filmmaker. I began with theater and storytelling but eventually was taken by individual people's life stories. For eleven years, my business was documentaries on personal histories for people in institutions. I got close to people's lives over generations, and I learned how a life is composed.

When you come to the bedside of somebody, it's one dot in the spectrum of his or her life. It's not "Oh, the sick person." It's this person's life story. At this point they might be sick, but I am already attuned to the larger life picture.

Part of what compassion is, is not seeing people in the small self of "the sick one" but in the larger self of the full trajectory of their life. The problem of being sick in the hospital is that your address is what your diagnosis is. You're the MS patient of this ward, the stroke victim on that ward. That smallness is devastating to the healing process. Compassion is walking in the room and seeing the larger self.

One of my earliest patients was my peer, in her forties. The cancer was distorting her whole body, a huge growth on her spine, and she was doubled over in a wheelchair. When I met her, she looked like she should have been dead a long time ago. I was surprised that she wasn't. The huge elephant in the room was that she wasn't mentioning death, dying, sickness, or anything. I let her set the agenda, and I realized she didn't want to talk about any of that. I saw her for a number of months, and death, dying, illness never came up. She'd talk about her cats. She wanted to know about my life.

She was going to be losing the ability to speak, yet she wasn't moving our time together towards any kind of spiritual discussion. But one day she took the straw from the water she was drinking and made a drop on one part of her leg and then another drop on the same leg and said, "This is me and this is Miriam" – her best friend, who had died. And then she smushed them together into one drop – at which point I used that as an entry point to say, "Are you afraid?"

"Yes," she responded.

"What are you afraid of?"

"How will it go? What's going to happen?"

She had a nurse who came in every day to tend to her body. I said, "Why don't you ask your nurse?"

She had a very peaceful conversation with Mary. "Will I be gasping? How will I stop breathing?" She was far away from talking about anything spiritual, but her fear was alleviated somewhat by hearing about what the process would be. So where my choice would have been to talk to her about soul and the afterlife, the lesson for me was that I had to meet her where she was. It was months before she did this little drawing and there was an inroad.

Each patient's story is amazing. Each person's death is as unique as his or her life. You leave at the threshold any expectations you have. You leave them at the door.

There is the Divine in the face of everybody whose path you cross. Sometimes I've wanted people not to suffer the way they did, but they had to die the way they had to die. That's always a lesson for me. I can't impose my vision to alter their path.

10

The Hospital as Village

Hospital nursing began making sense to me when I began to see the institution as a village.

This is perhaps imagination, but when you live your passions within the intelligence of imagination it can transform you. I invite the reader into the metaphor of the village because it's there that the vibrancy of compassion makes hospital work generous and true. It is here that this enviable vocation becomes the most visible.

My nursing career began outside of the hospital. For four years in Watsonville, California, I did home nursing, tending to Mildred, elderly and paralyzed. Without her ventilator Mildred would quickly die. Multiple sclerosis had completely compromised her ability to draw an independent breath.

I worked all night with Mildred, and occasionally on Sundays when she went to church, and sometimes during family get-togethers on the holidays. My work life drew me into the elemental poetry of being human – solitude and meditation through the night, on one hand, and small-town America on the other.

After Mildred it was Jesse Houts.

At fifteen years old, Jesse weighed forty-five pounds. Born with a rare non-progressive form of muscular dystrophy, Jesse had never walked. But he was an active teenager tooling around in his electric wheelchair with its ventilator breathing for him through a long blue tube connected to his tracheotomy.

Jesse was and is unsinkable. He'd faced death time and again – each time a rite of renewal for his appetite for life. Jesse took me into a village much different than the Republican Pentecostals of Mildred and her friends. With Jesse it was punk rock and anarchism. My efforts to get in touch with my inner teenager were, I think, more entertaining than pathetic. And to me, at least, more convincing than my inner Republican.

I was six years with Mildred and Jesse before I followed love to Los Angeles and entered into the world of hospitals.

After the intimacy of home care, UCLA Medical Center was intimidating – until I saw it as a village disguised as a hospital.

The village emerged out of the dark, slowly, as I learned my way around. "More miles of hallways than the Pentagon," a nurse supervisor told me.

Seeing my patients and their families through the village metaphor became the pleasure of the job.

Each of these souls became for me a citizen of a village world, or a visitor to it.

The village is divided into two communities, the patients and their families being one community and the staff being another. The two are completely interdependent, of course. They share a common desire that healing take place.

All know heartbreak and joy. Some are sick, and some very sick. Usually the sick ones are the patients.

But it's their common humanity that's the central point. That is what makes staff, patients, and their families a single village. It is also what makes compassion a possibility. The commonness of our humanity dispels alienation.

A village is a web of stories, each story a thread crossing other threads and making a pattern, a world of relationships. Doing home care with Mildred and Jesse, I became sensitive to the depth and breadth of stories that make up a single if "ordinary" life. At UCLA each patient's room, a nexus in the web where stories met, became a hut in the village, and the staff were like village healers, traveling from hut to hut.

The hospital has the hubbub of a village, lived in the flux of stories. There are the stories that patients tell their nurses, nurses tell their patients, patients tell each other, the employees tell one another, or a patient's mother tells you quietly in the hall. It's carnival one moment, a madhouse the next, yet quietly ordered, room by room, each hut in the village rich with its own stories.

Healthcare providers bear witness and participate in the "gathering of the clan" around the ill: family, church, friends, well-wishers. Indeed it *takes* a village to care for the ill.

The way of the Navajo people (the Diné) exemplifies this.

The Diné are culturally very different from their neighbors, the Hopi and the Zuni, whose ritual life circulates around the changes of season and the initiations of the boys and the girls. For the Navajo, the primary rituals are *singway* ceremonies, communal healing rites performed when someone is ill.

The patient goes to a diagnostician – a hand trembler, perhaps – who can say what brought on the illness and which *sing* would realign the patient with Spirit, clan, and the natural world.

Then the patient seeks out a *yathtali* (medicine man) to perform the ceremony.

A singway can last several nights and it benefits not only the sick one but whoever comes to the ceremony. It renews the tribe. It is, in fact, what binds Diné to Diné.

Everybody is accommodated, and a sheep is slaughtered so everyone has enough to eat.

In a village, every person has a place and everyone has a role. Author Michael Ventura tells an anecdote. He was teaching writing to teenagers and one of them stunned him with the statement: "Even a person in a coma has a purpose . . . because that person is being cared for by nurses, doctors, family and friends, and the purpose of all their lives is influenced and enhanced by caring for the person in the coma."

Once the hospital began to appear as a village, it was easy to see that the village metaphor extends beyond the hospital's doors.

The place of shared humanity *is* the village...

11

Grace and Graciousness

In Zimbabwe, when a stranger comes to the threshold of a village compound, he or she is brought water to drink even before being greeted. Every culture, perhaps every village, has its own forms of expressing grace and graciousness. Individuals have their own styles too. Rather a lot is conveyed by an authentic "welcome," by the simple gestures of receiving a guest. It is amazing how well this is communicated even across language barriers. The eloquence of silent gesture sometimes exceeds what might be said in words.

In the movie *The Doctor,* William Hurt plays a physician known for his cold efficiency who is diagnosed with cancer and so comes to "taste his own medicine." He learns what it is to be a nonentity hanging precariously from a diagnosis. At the end of the film he has his medical students admitted as patients for a day. Stripped, given gowns, asked those personal and sometimes humiliating questions, they are suddenly strangers in a domain most certainly not their own.

Healthcare workers often forget the vast distance between the patient's real life and the strange ways of hospital life.

Mr. Baxter and his family had been abducted into a sudden health crisis but had never really been received by the hospital.

He was a successful businessman in his late fifties who had merely a routine checkup with his private doctor. Completely without symptoms, his blood work was "strange," and imaging studies confirmed that he had extensive metastatic cancer.

Mr. Baxter was deep in a regimen of high-dose chemotherapy and had been lying in bed, unmoving and nonverbal, for a few days. The doctor's order was that every two hours artificial tears were to be instilled into his dry eyes. The chemo had rendered his kidneys nonfunctional so he was on dialysis.

Early in the shift, near midnight, his wife called. She was enraged, heartbroken, and confused.

"What are you doing to my husband? He was perfectly healthy before he went to Dr. Conrad! Our teenage kids are going out of their minds. We think Bill is going to die before he says good-bye."

I listened helplessly and then asked. "Do you want me to pray?"

"Would you?"

"I'd be honored."

When the shift quieted down I went into Mr. Baxter's room and sang and placed tears in his eyes. After I prayed aloud I said, "Mr. Baxter, your wife called an hour ago, and she and your kids are very concerned that you're going to leave this life without making any contact with them. It's a lot to ask, but could you possibly return?" I spoke to him father to father. Communicating with a father's heart was a way of gathering him into the circle of hospitality.

I couldn't know for sure if he understood, but his eyes welled up with what seemed more than the saline solution that I'd put in them.

The following afternoon I dropped into his room before my night shift began. Mr. Baxter was sitting up, looking dazed but alert as his wife fed him. He didn't recognize me, but his wife remembered my voice.

"Hi, Mr. Baxter. I was your nurse last night and have just come to see how you are doing."

"He prayed for you, Bill," his wife said.

I nodded that it was true. "I'm so glad to see you found your way back, Mr. Baxter."

"Yes. I was a long way from home," he said.

Receiving patients with the hospitality one would extend to a guest can be especially important across cultures, because for someone from another culture, the hospital is a foreign island in an already foreign land.

Mr. Ahmed was an elderly gentleman from Iraq admitted for chemotherapy for liver cancer. I had been warned that he was "a little paranoid," but chose to translate this as "a little fragile." Cancer and chemo can run anyone ragged.

Yes, paranoia was possibly a real concern. But I'd too often seen the tendency to let the previous shift's casual assessment color the way a patient is met and thereafter treated, perpetuating a relationship of I-It.

I poured some orange juice for Mr. Ahmed and his wife and greeted them with it. I make a point of meeting fragile patients last so I'm not distracted by the need to be elsewhere, and I knew from my experiences in the Arab world that the poetry of offering them juice as a first gesture would rhyme with the codes of hospitality they were familiar with.

Salaam aleikum, I said as I handed him the juice. Mr. Ahmed hesitated for a moment and then smiled and replied in perfect English, "And peace be with you as well."

Ice broken. Alliance made. His night was calm. The next night I brought a couple of bags of mint tea from home to greet him, remembering the syrupy sweetness of the mint tea in the Arab market of Jerusalem.

I was remembering also the exquisite hospitality of Muslim people. My wife and I were in Zimbabwe on September 11, 2001 and a few days later, flew with a couple of African friends to Mt. Sinai in Egypt to pray for peace. We were received with the generosity and solicitude that Arab people are famous for, and also with condolences for what had happened. Returning to America, I knew to honor Muslims because many Americans would simply be reactive from the terrible violence of 9/11.

One might say Mexico is closer to home than Iraq, but the distance between Mexico and a modern teaching hospital in Los Angeles can be culturally just as vast.

Mr. Ramirez, thirty-five years old, was dying. His kidneys were failing, and his cardiac monitor showed a grossly irregular heartbeat. The oxygen saturation level in his blood proved him on the edge of respiratory failure in spite of his face mask. Half a dozen family members had come from Mexico City and were holding vigil at his bedside.

In the midst of all this, his nurse Sharon was informed that the nurse supervisor insisted his room be vacated for a patient across the hall. Mr. Johnson was angry because he wanted a private room and Mr. Ramirez' room was the only one that could be made available. "Mexicans and their families," the charge nurse had whispered in exasperation.

Taking a few slow breaths and praying for skill, tact, and the right words, Sharon entered Mr. Johnson's room to appeal to him directly. She sympathized with his desire for a private room. "If I were a patient I'd want a room to myself as well."

"I explained to him the situation with Mr. Ramirez and then said, 'I've come to ask for a gesture of kindness on behalf of this family. He won't be around much longer, and I'm told there will be a discharge in the morning that will free up a room for you.' "

He was amenable. Sharon saw nothing of the combativeness and anger she'd been warned of. Mr. Johnson easily extended hospitality to another patient and his family.

We so often insist the patient accommodate to our world with all its institutionalized chaos but Sharon's conscription of Mr. Johnson into a small conspiracy showed how simple it can be to work from a more "hospitable" logic.

Hospitality to the patient, the patient's family and to the possibility of a death not transgressed.

Hospitality first and foremost to the spirit of kindness.

While there is a wide range of difference among European-Americans and also various degrees of assimilation among people of color, one way of understanding our variety is to look at how the question of "we-ness" is held. In the *whitened* space of hospital culture, families are sometimes received as intruders. As the stories of Messrs. Ahmed and Ramirez show, the village way of hospitality extends not only to the patient but also to the family and the culture. Disease, healing, and death exist in that deep context.

The next day I arrived at work early to meditate but after a while left the chapel to get some water and stretch my legs. In the lobby I came upon the Lakota healer Lone Eagle and his partner, Mourning Dove. Eagle's son David had been in a car accident and was in the emergency room. A poor man, Eagle was at the information desk trying to negotiate a minister's privilege of complimentary parking.

"I need to see your minister's credentials," the secretary said.

Eagle laid a small suitcase on her desk and opened it up, displaying a pouch of sacred tobacco, sage for smudging, a braid of sweet grass, his *chanupah* (pipe), and an eagle feather. "These are my credentials," he said. "I've come to do some doctoring on my son."

At this point I approached. "My name is Michael." I extended my hand. "I'll make the bridges for you in the ER. I'm a nurse here."

As we walked to ER I accidentally spilled much of my water. Eagle saw it as pouring a libation. "That water will bless our path," he said.

As we entered the extremely chaotic ER I clipped on my name tag, placed my stethoscope around my neck, and looked for the charge nurse. She immediately took me to be staff relief.

"Actually we have an unusual situation here," I explained.

David was wheeled out of CT scan a few minutes later, and Eagle, Dove, and I gathered around his gurney. Nurses, doctors, and other patients were exquisitely deferential. It was quiet enough to be a tipi on the plains as Eagle prayed in Lakota, feathered his son, and wept.

12

Conspiracies of Kindness

A hospital is a place where small conspiracies of kindness are always happening if you're alert enough to take note of them, consciously participate, or maybe even instigate.

These conspiracies are possible because, before anything else, a hospital is a field of interconnection. The staff knows this on the mundane level of the tasks they do in which they collectively sustain the lives of the ill.

Susan draws a couple of tubes of blood from Mrs. Goldwasser's central line at 4 a.m., careful not to awaken her. She asks a nurse's aide to take them to the lab. An hour later, the lab sends the message that the potassium level is dangerously low. With the weakness of her cardiac condition, this could provoke a fatal arrhythmia. She calls the doctor, who has her write an order for IV potassium, STAT. The secretary faxes the order to the pharmacy, and she picks up the med fifteen minutes later and hangs the IV to run over four hours. No need to wake the patient. She is sleeping like a baby.

A conspiracy of kindness. Susan, the nurse's aide, the lab, the doctor, the secretary, the pharmacy – all tending to a sleeping woman. One little conspiracy among many.

If a hospital is a web of stories, then we are a part of our patient's story and they a part of ours.

This is what makes the story of "conspiracy" possible.

Mrs. Goldwasser has a story. Susan knew just a bit of it. Her parents survived the Holocaust, and she told her of the insecurity that comes of being the daughter of survivors.

She knew a little of the stories of the secretary and the nurse's aide because she'd often worked alongside them. And also, the pharmacist. The young intern who prescribed the potassium she knew not at all, but was aware that we were all conspiring for Mrs. Goldwasser.

In Africa they say that every individual life is a story told by God, but the life of the village is told by the ancestors. There are always layers upon layers to our interweaving stories.

What brought Susan to the profession of taking care of the ill? What brought her to work this evening? What brought her to this little conspiracy of tending to this woman's sleep?

Healthcare providers can make use of the possibilities of conspiracy if they realize they are part of this web of stories, this field of interconnection.

It seems that patients are generally more aware that staff are participants in a story, their story, than the staff itself is. A cold nurse is immediately recognized as a cold nurse, a warm nurse as a warm one, and the theater of the day, or of the hospital stay, will play itself out accordingly.

Burnout among healthcare professionals is endemic because we flatten what we do of meaning. It becomes "just a job." We trivialize the work of our hands, do not recognize the web of interconnection we are a part of, or the conspiracies we might join on behalf of our patients or each other.

Sometimes it takes two to convey kindness to a frightened person.

Audrey was a black woman in her mid-forties with spinal cancer. She was on high-dose steroids to shrink her tumor, and the medication had made her emotionally unstable. In her eyes I was alternately a devil, a priest, or an angel. When she wasn't screaming, she had the sweetest, most luminous quality to her. The doctor wrote an order to place an indwelling catheter to drain her urine. By what grace might I be able to follow through on such an order?

As I was pondering this Art Patterson passed by her doorway. Art's a secretary, black, a Pentecostal, a good friend.

"Art my man, I need your help praying for somebody."

"Okay, Doggie Bones. Who needs praying?"

I tell him the situation and go get the catheter, and then we both came to her bedside.

"Audrey, this is my friend Art. I was telling him about how sick you've been feeling and asked him if he'd pray over you with me."

She settled into the calmest mood I'd seen her in as Art bathed her in the loving care of Jesus. And that mood lingered. After Art left, she received the catheter without the least resistance.

A third example of conspiracy.

Lucia barely arrived on the oncology floor when at the beginning of a shift, Dr. Wayne approached her to assist him and an intern in a procedure they were doing on Mrs. Otero, a needle biopsy of a rectal mass.

She greeted Mrs. Otero in Spanish while the doctor swabbed her for the biopsy. She could see she was frightened. Noting a cross around her neck, she began quietly singing an Ave Maria song that her mother taught her as a girl while the doctor injected the lidocaine.

Ave Maria. Dios te salve, María, llena eres de gracia, el Señor es contigo. Bendita tú eres entre todas las mujeres, y bendito es el fruto de tu vientre, Jesús. Santa María, Madre de Dios, ruega por nosotros, pecadores, ahora y en la hora de nuestra muerte. Amen ...

"Let the song carry you, Mrs. Otero. Let Maria hold you," Lucia said softly and ran her fingers through her hair. "She shifted from being a frightened and physically tight woman and relaxed into the song. I encouraged her to breathe deeply, and when the biopsy was done, I set off to begin my shift."

A few minutes later Dr. Wayne again approached her in the hall. "Could you come back to room 1018? We need another specimen from Mrs. Otero."

"I sometimes sing to patients to make procedures easier for them, but this was the first time I'd done so in front of doctors. Initially, there had been the clinical distance that sometimes accompanies a rectal biopsy, and now there was a warmth."

Santa María, Madre de Dios, ruega por nosotros, pecadores, ahora y en la hora de nuestra muerte. Amen ...

13

Smuggling Beauty

Peacemaker and author Anne Herbert advocated practicing "random kindness and senseless acts of beauty" in response to the random violence and senseless acts of terror that pervade the daily news. From the perspective of its most defenseless patients, a hospital is not without its acts of random violence. People arrive stressed and the hospital can push them further. This is true for staff as well as patients.

There is a modest power to the random act of kindness that greatly outweighs the smallness of the gesture – an unexpected reminder that beauty exists when the world itself seems to be fading into the distance. Beauty is a salve for a fragmented world, a gift to the giver as well as the receiver. And being surprised by beauty is also a gift. I remember such moments for years on end. An orchid, green-veined, left at the nurses station by a patient's husband. The fragrance of a bearded iris on a bedside table. Packing an old man's bedsore with saline gauze while an elephant birthed on television. Cupping a yellow and black spider in my hand to deliver outside to the flowers. Or just the light that rises in anyone's face when they feel recognized and connected with. Beauty is an oasis. In it is found replenishment.

Smuggling beauty to vulnerable patients often requires small conspiracies.

"The only way to learn Romanian is in bed," said Sylvia, my Romanian nurse's aide.

"For God's sake, Sylvia, I don't want to learn Romanian. I just want you to translate a few lines. And please don't make them too sexy. It's a quote from the Koran. And besides, the patient is eighty-five years old. And demented. Like you."

"Pot calling the kettle black," she sniffed. "Okay. What is it?"

"If I had but three loaves of bread, I'd sell one and buy hyacinths, for they would feed my soul."

"What? That's not sexy? And why do you want to give the Koran to an old Romanian? Is she a Muslim? There are no Muslims in Romania, I can tell you that."

"No, she's Catholic. And out of her mind and lonely. She could use a little beauty."

"Hyacinths?"

"Almost."

Sylvia translated the Koran and I transcribed it onto a Styrofoam cup. I'd pilfered some flowers from the chapel and went to Mrs. Codrescu's room on the fifth floor. I'd admitted Mrs. Codrescu the previous night. Intractable nausea and change of consciousness. Her daughter nervously left her mom behind, nervous because mom was so confused and didn't speak a word of English. I wanted to leave the flowers for her daughter as much as for Mrs. Codrescu so she knew someone had an eye on her mother.

When I arrived in her room with my little bouquet – feeling, I confess, like a paramour – I was surprised to find her gone.

I went to the nurse's station and asked the secretary, "What happened to the Romanian woman in 545?"

"Romanian?" replied Donna. "I don't know nothing about no Romanian."

I paused and re-gathered. "Do you have any lonely, really screwed up patients who might like a flower?" I decided it best not to mention the Romanian Koran.

"Lots. Lots and lots. What kind you'd like? There's a Mexican woman in 516. She's completely nuts."

"Thanks."

As I approached 516 I was hoping the patient was asleep. My Spanish is not good enough to explain why a strange white guy with a stethoscope felt compelled at 5 a.m. to bring a flower in a cup inscribed in a language which he did not know. The woman could simply wake up to the mystery of it. And the beauty. The message in Romanian wouldn't matter. Flowers have a beauty everyone recognizes.

Sometimes serendipity just happens. The Mexican woman in 516 turned out, in fact, to be Mrs. Codrescu – alert, not the least agitated, looking as if she'd been expecting me. Raising my finger to my lips and handing her my gift, I pointed at the Koranic verses and nodded my head as she read them. My role was simple: The village idiot had arrived. Her smile was simplicity itself.

I had searched the web looking for different flower poems. No luck. All so sappy and sentimental, sub-Hallmark. Japanese poetry had possibilities, but I loved the body and meaning of the Koran, and so it found itself at the bedside table of many patients, some that I knew, some I didn't. Co-workers were happy to translate. I even had the hyacinth poem translated into contemporary Arabic for an Egyptian gentleman on the oncology floor.

I don't remember when it was that I started smuggling beauty into the hospital – as much for myself as for the patients. I'd do it for the sheer pleasure in a sometimes harsh work life. Sometimes I'd just sing. Once, while walking the hallways down to the pharmacy to get a medication, I passed a room where someone was crying out. She was an old black woman and not entirely coherent. I paused for just a moment to sing her one of the Yoruba sacred songs I know, and to whisper that it's all right. And for a moment it was, the way beauty sometimes makes things, all right for a moment.

And then there were the Braille origami cranes. A blind Japanese woman, Mrs., Yasu, grateful for the care she received at UCLA, made hundreds of cranes out of Braille paper as benedictions for the health of fellow patients. The chaplaincy would leave a couple of dozen a week in the chapel. At the beginning of my work week, I'd take a few and keep my eyes peeled for who I could pass this woman's gift on to.

Marsha was an attractive forty-five-year-old professional woman and a stone cold alcoholic. She had finally put the bottle down and was admitted with extreme withdrawal – delirium tremens, the proverbial snakes crawling up her legs. I was her nurse for all of four hours before I was floated to another floor, another bunch of patients. A nurse's aide was scheduled to sit at her bedside through the night so she wouldn't harm herself. Her wrists and ankles were fastened to the bed with four-point restraints.

"Untie me! Untie me! Get me out of here. I demand you set me free! You can't do this! You can't!" It wasn't at all clear that she knew she was in a hospital or why she should be.

"I wish I could untie you but I can't. I know this must be humiliating, but you're withdrawing from alcohol and if I undo you, you might hurt yourself."

She paused. It was clear that she didn't know or had forgotten that she was crazed from lack of liquor. "Screw you! Release me. I will sue you. You'll see. I need to urinate."

"I'll get you a bed pan."

"No. Untie me!"

And on and on.

The doctor wrote one of those impossible orders. "Foley catheter to gravity" to drain her bladder of urine. This would mean having two strong people pry her legs open while I swabbed her with betadine, dipped the catheter tip in surgical gel, spread her labia with my free hand, and inserted the cath into the urethra of this writhing, angry woman.

Sterilely.

Right. Sure. Done it before. But in Marsha's case I decided it would be less denigrating to convince her of the virtues of the bedpan or to clean her up after she soiled herself.

Before heading off to the other floor, I reported off to my replacement, sheepishly explaining why I didn't place the catheter. No nurse likes to leave "dirty work" for the new shift, but Anne understood that this woman was in no frame of mind for such a procedure.

I returned briefly to Marsha's room at 6 a.m. with my little Braille crane and the well-used wisdom from the Koran. She looked truly ragged, but the first wave of DTs had softened. Her hands and feet were untied, and I helped her up to the bedside commode.

When she finished I gave her the origami.

"I brought you this because I'm so moved by your courage. Dropping the alcohol may be the bravest thing you've ever done. This was made by a blind patient for other patients. You'll find your way through the dark. There is a life on the other side of hell. Thank you for teaching me about courage."

"Thank you, thank you," she said a couple dozen times amid gales of laughter. I spent just a few minutes with her because I had to return to the floor I was working.

Mr. Hewitt was a financial consultant in his late fifties, a man of great character and presence. A mistake had been made – I don't remember what – but the hospital had almost killed him. He was coded and brought back and so had an intimate knowledge of his mortality. I asked him, "What is it to live with death over your left shoulder all the time?" He'd also had a heart transplant a few years earlier – and was much concerned about matters of the heart. At 1 a.m. he called me into his room.

"I've been tossing and turning for hours. I can't get my son out of my mind. He's 17 years old. What can I offer him now? He's being taken by the materialism of the culture, and I'm afraid he's going to give his life to that nonsense."

Listening to Mr. Hewitt I felt that thick, fatherly helplessness before a teenager – my own – before the anger and sense of futility of a friend's son, my father's when I was 17 and homeless. Helplessness seems woven into the vulnerable truths of fathers and sons. This helplessness is stretched by the knowledge, no, the blues song, of the ordeal we've gone through ourselves to become men. And *that* we are just beginning to digest.

Not knowing what to say, I started with what I was sure of. "You know," I attempted, "after my fortieth birthday I went into the forest for a few months to pray and meditate. After a couple of months of sitting still, I began to hear the murmur of my mother's prayers that have sustained me through some very dark times. They were almost audible. I certainly couldn't hear them when I was homeless - I was so full of my passion and desperation. It's strange what passes from generation to generation and how it passes. My grandfather I despised until a few years before his death, when I saw what a remarkable man he was. And my father - well, we got close only after his death."

"So you're saying I should trust the light that's in him and live by the values that I have suffered to understand - and somehow this is passed on to him? By what - osmosis?"

"Somehow passed on. Or not," I replied. "That's the rub, the helplessness. Your spirit is with him and will persist after you're gone. You're in him. But you remember well what it took to get real with what's in you. All you're left with is being faithful to your own soul and believing in him until he believes in himself."

An hour after he fell asleep, I admitted a new patient to the adjacent bed. His roommate was thirty-five, homeless, with a nasty, oozing cellulitis on his left calf. He was in a lot of pain, and so I kept him still with morphine. It was January and we talked about being homeless.

"Damn it gets cold this time of year," I said. "Cold and lonely."

"You got that right, brother."

As the sun rose both of them were sleeping, I left a Braille crane on Mr. Hewitt's bedside table with a note: "This is for your son and for whatever dark passage he must walk learning to be a man. Live by the best of who you are. Seek his light and praise it. Blessings."

I signed it "Michael," with my address.

I received a letter from him a couple of weeks later:

Dear Michael,
I wanted to thank you so much for your gift to my son. I wept as I ran my inadequate fingers across the symbols that have given sight to so many. Those without sight must see so much more.

I put the origami in a box with your note and a note to my son. Basically I told him in the letter that when he feels his anger take over, to reach into the box very gently and retrieve this remarkable work of art and heart. Close his eyes and gently rub his fingers across this tremendous accomplishment and think of how you would have to be at peace with yourself to complete such arduous work.

When we were kids, my sisters and I used to make up words to describe my dad. One of the words was "wisdomious," defined as "one having done deeds which took wisdom." One cannot always be right – unless of course you're my dad. If you think about the heart of a person and not so much as what comes out of his mouth, you would see that all he wanted was to be perfect in his son's eyes.

I put together socks, razors and other essential in a box for Keith, the homeless man I met in the hospital. My son and I are meeting him on Saturday so that my son can experience the pain and degradation of those who pine their existence.

Warmest personal regards,
Lew Hewitt

This is quintessential conspiracy – the gentle power of these origami cranes quietly threading healing beauty and goodwill from patient to patient without the patients ever meeting, or me even meeting the maker of the cranes.

We can all do good to others this way – just send it out, like the Japanese woman did.

14

Finding Beauty in Unexpected Places

Sometimes one finds beauty in the oddest places.

The dungeon, for example.

I met Jake suddenly, very suddenly. As a nursing student, part of my psych training entailed spending two weeks in the "dungeon." One South, San Jose Valley Medical Center.

Aptly named, the dungeon was a locked ward for people bursting in full psychosis: off the streets and put in the dungeon for three days, or two weeks, until they were "controlled on meds."

I met Jake in a little niche, for the moment just the two of us. Perhaps five foot five inches, fading blue tattoos, a mass of muscle and fat. His skin was the color of a man who might well have been in the dungeon for decades. His face was a mask of violence.

Without saying a thing he quickly cornered me, grabbed my collar, and pinned me against the wall. Looking in my eyes he said, "You know I could take your neck and twist it and that would be the end of you."

"You could for sure, but I kind of hope you don't."

"Hell, man. I'm not going to do that. You think I'd do that to you? I like you. Let's go hang out with the others."

The others were Jake's *posse*, folks he knew from previous recyclings through the dungeon. Awkwardly settling into their company I soon found I could trust these patients who dared relate to me as peer. After shooting the bull for half an hour, one of them, young Jim, said, "Have you ever been suicidal? Are you now suicidal? Have you considered the method by which you will kill yourself?"

I was startled and stammered to find honest answers. Jake and Jim started laughing and then it dawned that I was being received as an honorary madman through the rites of humiliation every psych patient knows by heart. They were enjoying admitting to the dungeon this madman who was posing as a nursing student.

Through the years of my nursing career, every time I have asked a crazed patient these obligatory questions, I've remembered hanging out with my *posse* and inwardly smile. Often the preface was "forgive me these questions are required" or, if the patient was clearly suicidal, "this is the hospital's effort to take care of you."

Once in a teaching hospital, I was admitting a woman who was depressed. Kim lost three friends to drive-by shootings. After asking her how she might want to kill herself, I was to have her sign a consent or refusal to take an experimental medication.

Soon the two of us were laughing uproariously at the mind that thought it plausible to greet patients, many in abject states of paranoia, with the choice to be or not to be a guinea pig. The heart is eclipsed behind such questions. They speak from a bureaucratic soul and create the widest possible distance between a person in crisis and the institution that strips them further of power.

In the village that I serve the mad are honored guests not to be approached crudely. There is a finesse to translating bureaucratic protocol into human graciousness and the guinea pig gambit was crude beyond telling.

Jake had been a Marine in Vietnam and had been in and out of facilities since the war. The staff knew him as a "frequent flyer" – he couldn't keep away. He'd been discharged just the previous week but was soon rearrested – he'd broken into a nice car near a public park and torn up its dashboard while screaming obscenities and acting psychotic. The dungeon was home for Jake. "People are real here," he explained.

The second week in the dungeon, Jake almost completely ignored me and everybody else too except for Mabel. Mabel was a woman in her seventies who was going through electroshock therapy for catatonia. Jake took Mabel under his wing. "She's my mom's age," he said.

Mabel was nonverbal. After her electroshock treatment, Jake wheeled her around in her wheelchair to watch the birds outside, few that there were. He put three stellar blue feathers of a jay into her limp hands. As they watched other patients play basketball he'd dab her drool with Kleenex he'd brought for the occasion. By nursing standards he was impeccable. Could it be that Jake was in part compelled to return to the dungeon because love was possible there?

The neuro floor at UCLA Medical Center is as mysterious as the dungeon and sometimes as harsh.

I admitted Katyn for a thorough work-up for her seizure activity. She'd had seizures for only a few years, ever since she went to Morocco for the village festivities of Joujouka. The villagers there, as Muslims, celebrate the rites of the god Pan, and have done so since the times of the Roman Empire.

"Joujouka? Pan? Did you know Pan is the god of epilepsy?"

She admitted she didn't while I hooked her up to her conehead Buck Rodgers headgear so a monitor tech could watch her brain waves on a television screen alongside a dozen screens with other brainwaves zigzagging across them.

The next day she and her roommate Lisa, a young mute black woman, also an epileptic, were both deprived of sleep to see if sleeplessness might provoke a seizure that could be monitored and studied. It turns out Katyn was a virtuoso at American Sign Language and a performance artist. They put a cassette of gospel music on the table between their beds and sat facing each other, their hands dancing the lyrics as their brain waves danced in the monitor room.

"You call Spirit like this, and you're gonna get your seizures in no time," I called from the hallway.

This silent call and response praising God was performance art spontaneous and indescribably beautiful.

Mr. Ralph, age sixty-one, had arrived in the cardiac unit either to die or to get a new heart. Everyone had assured him a new heart was the thing, but he wasn't entirely convinced. He was very tired, and death did have its virtues. Nevertheless, a new heart, harvested from the chest of a thirty-seven-year-old stranger found its way into his chest. From our first conversation he spoke of gratitude, grief, joy – and befuddlement. He was feeling things for the first time.

"I never weep. Never. But now I weep all the time. I was a first-class bastard. Now I'm feeling compassion."

Mr. Ralph had recently retired from the CIA because of his heart condition. Thirty years "on company business," first in Southeast Asia, then the Congo, and finally Central America in the eighties. As he talked about Central America I saw that some of his tears were bitter.

"I was in El Salvador briefly in 1987," I ventured, remembering the fear in the air and the blood on the ground. "And then I went to Nicaragua."

"It was an ugly scene," he said. "Very ugly. If Americans only knew what their country does to the world. I have witnessed, and done, horrible things. El Salvador 1987. Aye!"

Another aspect of his newfound compassion showed itself the following day. His roommate, who happened to be a thirty-seven-year-old man, had just been discharged. Mr. Reyes was on the short list for a new heart and had to go through various pre-transplant tests. He went home to await the phone call that would inform him his turn had come.

"I guess I became a father figure. Or a brother or something. Our hearts are the same age!" The two men were rapt in conversation before Mr. Reyes left the hospital, Mr. Ralph counseling the young man and talking about how the new heart changed his life.

Sometimes you smuggle beauty. And sometimes beauty just grabs you by the scruff of the neck and takes you. These patients, each facing the unimaginable, revealed beauty where we might least expect to find it: Mad Jake adopting mad Mabel like a dutiful son, two epileptic patients silently belting out gospel, the CIA agent discovering the gift of tears.

When beauty bears a human face, we become beauty, don't we?

15

The Illness Runs through Everybody

Conversation with Robert Carroll, MD

Among many traditional people – the Navajo for example, or the Shona people of Africa – it is understood that illness pulls the soul away from an ordered life, thins out its relationships with the world. Healing ceremonies thus reestablish relationship with the world. In the hospital this happens when the loving family or group of church members gathers at a bedside to pray. Psychiatrist Dr. Robert Carroll understands this truth and works with it in his practice. He also brings beauty to the ill and the dying and evokes it from them in his work with poetry therapy.

Michael: What called you to the profession of psychiatry?

Robert: I was inspired to go into psychiatry as a medical student. The doctor goes on rounds with the chief resident, followed by the first year resident, followed by the intern, followed by the medical students: little ducks in a row. And they walk into a room, and the doctor says, yes, we have to take off your breast, you have a cancer, I'll see you in the morning, and walks out. I being the littlest duck would always be the person who stayed with the patient and see what he or she was going through. When I finished medical school. I decided I wanted to solidify my skills as a physician, so I did a year of internal medicine. But then, having become a competent physician, I felt free to go into psychiatry. It was the only specialty for which you were paid for spending time with people.

Michael: But you nonetheless work often with people who are physically ill.

Robert: Oh, yes. Over the course of my work as a psychiatrist I've dealt with a number of people who were physically ill and having psychiatric difficulties. One case in particular was a thirty-two-year-old woman with terminal lung fibrosis. She and her husband had a child with cerebral palsy, and she hadn't bonded to the child because she'd been in the hospital for numerous operations. She was in so much pain that she tried to kill herself with the complicity of her husband, who didn't want her to die but wanted to honor her wishes.

The attempt failed. Her husband could no longer abide that and took her medications away, and without her medications she didn't know what to do. And so they were referred to me to see whether there was anything I could offer.

With that patient and her husband, and the two-year-old daughter I facilitated a healing among the family members. Even though she died within a year, the family was able to carry on afterwards. I was flying by the seat of my pants the whole way. At the same time, my father was in his three-year terminal demise from diabetic multi-systems failure. And I had an accident where I had to have knee reconstruction. All of those things happening at once made me feel quite overwhelmed and I was looking for a way to deal with that.

Michael: I hear this story often: the pivotal patient who pushes us to the edge of what we know, coupled sometimes with personal crises. A very intense season of learning about human suffering. How did you make sense of it?

Robert: Well, the typical way that a psychiatrist would do that probably is to go into therapy, but it's not what I wanted to do. I decided that I'd try to write my experience as a way of making it real. I started writing that and other stories about illness and healing and death and dying.

During the course of the next several years that I wrote these pieces, I'd present them publicly at conferences, grand rounds at the hospital, church groups, wherever. Once I read my poetry into the service at the church, and it was a way of facilitating a dialogue among congregants who had lost members of their family. What I found was the people were responding to the work, not necessarily because they thought it was wonderful poetry, but because there was something about my personal experience which touched a universal nerve.

One day I was in Santa Barbara doing a presentation at grand rounds at Cottage Hospital. Afterward, a woman in the audience asked me if I'd ever heard of poetry therapy. She explained that poetry therapy was the use of poetry and literature, both written and spoken language, in the service of healing, growth, and transformation. I came to understand that a lot of people were actually engaged in the very kind of thing I was involved in. They were in an association called the National Association for Poetry Therapy. And so I hooked up with them.

Michael: So your personal crisis brought you into a deeper understanding of healing?

Robert: Yes. What I believe is that the writing and reading of poetry taps into natural healing processes that we all have. If I ask an audience, "Who here among you are poets?" maybe a few people would raise their hands. If I ask them, "How many of you have written poems?" maybe twenty percent will raise their hands. If I ask, "How many of you have ever written a poem or used a poem in a time of need?" most people will raise their hands. And when you go around and have people report on when they did that, almost invariably they did it in a very natural way. They needed to do it. They were called to it. What is most personal is most universal.

There are two ways that physicians deal with patients. One is technical, and the other is personal. There are a lot of physicians who are technically proficient, they may be able to take out the tumor and all of the rest, but personally they really are cut off.

I did an ad hoc study many years ago in which I interviewed physicians who had developed major serious illnesses. I wanted to see what the effect was of going from the doctor's side of the bed to the patient's side of the bed. What they all uniformly reported was that they used to feel they understood what their patients were talking about and now they knew they didn't. They may still not know what the patients are talking about. but at least they know that they don't know what they're talking about.

While we have a professional relationship to what we do, we also have a personal relationship to what we do. And I believe that the professional has to be ministered through the personal. There has to be a way of delivering one's expertise in an interpersonally alive way for the possibility of healing to occur.

Michael: What is healing really about anyway?

Robert: Healing is not just about getting rid of the tumor or reversing the pulmonary fibrosis, it's also about healing the person in their role in the family, in society, and in the culture at large. And it's about healing the rifts that occur, because any serious illness runs through everybody. So the healing part of what I do is to work with people in the context in which they live and in their relationships they have with their committed family members.

The disease is the breakdown in the body – the tumor, the infection – but the illness is the way the person brings that disease into their life, into the world, and into their relationships. So the person can have a very bad disease but not be that ill. Or they can have pretty minimal disease and be very ill, in terms of how they relate to others.

Michael: How do you use poetry in your practice?

Robert: When somebody comes in to see me, I do an intake evaluation, and then I will typically ask them if they ever do any writing. A lot of people I see keep a journal or have written poetry. I encourage them to bring their journals or to bring their poetry or to write something in the service of what we're doing or to explore something. I might give them an assignment or make a suggestion.

For example, if someone writes a piece in the third person, I might ask them to put it in the first person so they can pass the meaning of the piece through themselves more directly. One woman wrote a journal entry about a visit her younger sister made to her. On the way back to the airport after the visit she kept looking over at the sister and wrote all the associations about their life together. Many of them were critical of her sister. As a writing exercise I asked her to write the same piece from the point of view of her sister looking at my patient sitting in the driver's seat as she was being driven to the airport. It's amazing the honesty and focus people bring to their writing.

When I do public talks on writing and healing, usually I'll introduce poems. For example, I might read a poem by Rilke, called "Breakthrough."

> *Sometimes I feel I'm pushing through solid rock alone.*
> *Everything close is close to my face,*
> *and everything close to my face is stone.*
> *I have no experience in this grieving.*
> *So these things make me feel small.*
> *You be the master and break through,*
> *then your great transforming will happen to me,*
> *and my great grief cry will happen to you.*

I'll present that poem, maybe I'll put it on the screen or handout, and I'll ask people if there is any line in there that they relate to, or that they think is important, or that they don't like. How do they relate to that poem? People will always say, "I really like that." "Wow, breakthrough, that was great." Or "pushing through solid rock – yeah, I get claustrophobic."

Whatever it is that comes out of the group I will assign a writing exercise, like "Remember a time when you felt you were pushing through solid rock? Or a time when you felt alone? See the scene. What are the smells, the sounds, the feel of the air?" When the participants read what they've written to the group, I'll ask people to write down any line that strikes them from what others have written, and then use those lines as clues to the healing they themselves need. The clues are in the resonance between their stories and the stories other people tell. This is what makes the personal universal.

A friend of mine, Kykosa Kajangu, from the Congo, has collected proverbs from a number of African tribes. These proverbs are the way cultural wisdom is handed from generation to generation. Kykosa has combined and fashioned many of these into poems on Friendship, Love, Death, Illness, and so on. He calls this writing "Wisdom Poetry." He and I and another friend, the poet/physician Dr. Jack Coulehan have presented to inspire participants to write their own wisdom poetry in the service of transformation.

Here's one of the poems I read.

It's called *Being the Stone:*

> *I want to be the stone and tell*
> *how she held me*
> *in the palm of her hand*
> *rolled me between her fingers*
> *slipped me into her mouth*
> *tasted my salt*
> *tumbled me around*
> *Then she ran her tongue along my edge*
> *and rubbed my cool body across the scar*
> *of her breast*
> *put me in her pocket*
> *took me home*
> *gave me to her daughter –*
> *a special gift*

Most poetry therapists work in groups, so they will bring poems that are relevant to a particular group, like substance abuse groups. They'll bring poems that were written by addicts. Grieving groups write poems about grief, courage, and carrying on.

Michael: Tell me about the work you were involved with about poetry and brain cancer.

Robert: In a particular project at UCLA, I was asked to assign six poets to six patients with brain cancer and have the poets help the patients find the words to express their experience. The poetry opened people's eyes because they came to understand things about brain cancer patients which are not always so apparent. Because when people get a diagnosis like brain cancer it's like, "Oh, my God, it's all downhill and I'll die." And it's true.

In general, they do die. Yet people go through amazing changes when they realize they have limited time.

One woman, when she found out she had brain cancer, said that she had always wanted to go to Rwanda to see the gorillas. So she went to Rwanda with her husband, and they trekked up the mountains through the jungle towards the gorillas, and she wasn't making it. The guide said, "Well, I'll try to convince her to go back," but she insisted on going on. And then at some point she just couldn't go on, and she lay down in the grass, and the gorillas came out of the jungle to her.

We have had people say that if they had everything to consider and do it all over again, they wouldn't change anything because of what they learned. It's not like everybody would wish that, but there is something that you learn from the experience of being ill.

16

Beatitude, Death, and the Mother of Beauty

Over thirty years ago, Elizabeth Kubler-Ross had just come out with her seminal work, *Death and Dying*. Classes were being taught in colleges and universities. Some of us – myself for example – imagined a transformation of the culture's naïve and brutal relationship with the simple fact of mortality and bereavement. I remember being taken by the simple Latin words, *ars moriendi*, the medieval "art of dying" that once had a place in European culture. Could we not re-imagine such an art for the contemporary world?

Of course the pathological denial of death persists, distorting the culture from the intimacy of personal and family choices to the warp of avoidances in medical institutions. The craft of compassion must walk in the valley of the denial of death skillfully and with generosity. We are a frightened lot, we humans, and we can only honor our frailty.

An uncanny silent awareness in people accompanies those souls that are getting ready for death. Days of being lost, quiet, in some far interior place, but also a knowing.

I took care of Mrs. Serbanescu three years before she died at 90 – an incompetent nurse's aide in a dingy little nursing home. Our conversations were always the same: halved.

The first half: "I want to die. Kill me please. Please kill me. I can't live here. This is horrible. Can't you kill me?"

"It is horrible," I would respond. "I am so sorry that your life's come to this. But I can't kill you, dear. I really can't, though I know it'd make you very happy. I'd lose my job for sure."

Every day we'd laugh at that one and then shift the conversation to the second half: our shared passion, Romanian music. I'd recently gotten quite fanatic about the cimbalom and what Gheorghe Zamfir does on the pan pipes. Not to mention the gypsy music.

"Gypsy music?" She was intrigued. The gypsies were despised when she was a girl but so alive for her. Sometimes she'd get a little flirtatious when we talked about their music.

And so it was day after day.

I never did say goodbye to Mrs. Serbanescu, but during second semester of nursing school Mrs. Serbanescu was admitted from the convalescent home to the small community hospital where I was doing a clinical rotation. She'd had a silent heart attack and was unresponsive on arrival.

I came to visit her one evening after my school week ended, sat at her bedside and said, "Mrs. Serbanescu? It's Michael. Do you remember me? It's been a long time since we've talked like we used to. Remember? We talked music, gypsy music. The violin, Mrs. Serbanescu. Do you remember the violin?"

I talked this way for perhaps twenty minutes. It had been a week and a half since she had said a word or opened her eyes. She just lay on her back and breathed. But she did open her eyes and said, "I remember you," closed her eyes and returned to just breathing.

Back at the hospital on Monday I wasn't assigned Mrs. Serbanescu by my professor, but I quietly entered her room just to see how she was.

An uncanny silent awareness is in people who are getting ready to die, a knowing even at the threshold. I was in the room not a minute when she expired her last breath. It was clear that she had waited for me or perhaps merely felt my presence enter the room. She knew it was time to let go.

How? I can't say. But it was transparently evident that she *knew*.

Her death fell lighter than a feather. I'd not seen the face of death before, and I saw it then in its most benevolent form, its beatitude.

"Death is the mother of Beauty, " writes Wallace Stevens, "hence from her, Alone, shall come fulfillment to our dreams. And our desires."

There are those who wait and those who don't. The same uncanny awareness pertains. June BlueSpruce tells the story of a beloved grandmother with brain cancer, shaved head, obese or perhaps bloated by her medications. "I spent a lot of time turning her over in bed, bathing her. She was comatose."

"There was a lot of chatter over her body and I know that the last sense to go is hearing. I insisted that people be present to the patient. I was thought of as strange."

Her family was anguished that she was dying and didn't want to let her go. "When I'd come into her room I'd whisper in her ear, 'You can go now. They'll be fine. It's all right.' She died within twenty-four hours."

They do listen, the dying. Sometimes Dina would take her early morning break in the rooms of patients who were in the long process of letting go to death.

"Sometimes there is no family. Nobody should die alone, but people do often enough – the body still and cold for 4 a.m. vitals, the last breath unwitnessed," she told me. Sitting vigil on behalf of a family that does not exist or is disengaged – here at this most sacred of moments the village becomes very real. Here Dina would extend presence as she hoped it would be extended to her when that day comes. The village that is the human community rests on this small, silent choice.

Dina didn't know Mr. Ortega. His was another nurse. She only knew that he was very ill, on a cardiac monitor, and in an isolation room because of antibiotic resistant bacteria. And that he had an order: Do not resuscitate. She put on her isolation get-up and came in and introduced herself.

"I'm just going to sit quietly by your bedside and pray. Pray and be silent."

She sat silently for half an hour and then said, "Mr. Ortega, I want you to know that I'm aware it's been a long hard road that brought you to this point. If you feel death coming, you can give yourself to it. It's really okay." Then she returned to silence.

Twenty minutes later his nurse arrived. The cardiac monitor at the nurse's station relayed what she already knew. Mr. Ortega was flat line.

When this happened with a second patient the following week on the same floor, Dina was sure somebody would take her for a homicidal nurse.

It seems to me that with these three patients there was, again, some uncanny communication soul to soul. And that there is an etiquette to releasing people from the costume of mortal flesh. Yet often the long lingering between worlds awaits this simple permission, the simple statement that letting go is the most trustworthy of acts. "If I were dying, would I want someone to say 'It's okay to let go?' " asked Dina.

"I probably would."

And then there's that other invisible process that happens at the edge of death. I saw it most vividly when my friend Helene was dying at home. There were half a dozen of us holding vigil through the night. Her young lover, Jill, approached me about how these things go.

I said, "Well, it's like a slipknot. The dying person pulls at one end of the thread, and all of us pull at the other. Letting go happens from both ends. And then there's when the knot unties, always at exactly the right moment. Don't expect death to be necessarily dramatic. It can be very quiet."

Helene's death was not dramatic, but it did have a flair to it. My wife and I were awakened by some commotion and leaped up to her bedside to see her recumbent body sit bolt upright and then collapse in her son's arms. I mean, the woman had style.

One can never overestimate the ministry of the dying, even of the dead, for it is a true ministry. Helene's son had had a bitter relationship with his mother several decades thick. Not one given to sentiment, he told me, "Most all of that is healed now. It healed the moment she died in my arms." All of us who witnessed it were likewise changed by the presence of a good death.

The shift is over, and I stop by Maggie's room. Maggie died just an hour ago at age one hundred and five. She practiced as a pediatrician into her nineties. "I told my daughters to keep an eye on me just in case I start losing it, you know what I mean?" she'd explained to me.

Even after her death she carried the good-humored dignity that had made her such an attractive person. I closed her eyes and whispered a Hail Mary. "Now and at the hour of our death. Amen." She was Catholic.

"If you see a bright light, Maggie, move towards it. I know it is too bright at first, but you will get used to it. That is the way of freedom."

Then I kissed her forehead and said, "Go well, Maggie. You made it."

Step Three

Radical Empathy

About Radical Empathy

Dakshen nyamje is translated as "equalizing and exchanging self and other," It's unfortunate that when one names such an experience in Tibetan it's instantly rendered impenetrable. *Dakshen nyamje* resonates with the Cherokee proverb: "You can only understand somebody else if you've walked two moons in their moccasins."

"Exchanging" is that simple and that essential. Sometimes *tonglen* gives way to "exchanging." With Jimmy, after an hour of "breathing in," his face distorted by the extremity of his anguish, "breathing out" the freshness of loving-kindness, we were quite "exchanged." "Exchanging" is an amalgam of complete equality and unimpeded empathy. "Exchanging" is not possible when one indulges thoughts of being superior. Our stories of sorrow and joy imprint the passage of moons from which we empathize with another's sorrow and joy.

Step Three is about the activity of compassion that proceeds from that wisdom and about the wisdom of humility before those who are suffering what we cannot comprehend. Radical empathy follows through on the question, "what if it were me or someone close to me who is suffering so?"

Amber is twenty-five and has leukemia. She loves the theater and at her bedside there is a photo of her in *A Midsummer Night's Dream*. For the moment she's undone by a stem cell transplant, her gums bleeding, asleep on Ativan. My daughter is Amber's age and I whisper this to her father when I bring him a cup of coffee. A swift, silent understanding. Nothing more need be said. This is *radical empathy*.

Mrs. Brown just had a mastectomy, as had my wife, and she is painfully self-conscious of her flat left side. Such was the rapport between us that I borrowed from my love of my wife's beauty. I laughed, "The running joke with my wife is that women with two breasts have come to look a little unnatural to me." Mrs. Brown confessed that she seemed to have more trouble with her mastectomy than her husband. "Borrowing from my wife's beauty" was *radical empathy*.

Here we cross the boundary towards *living* compassion. I try not to overuse the word "epistemology" because it makes this undereducated fool look so much more intelligent than' he actually is. Yet there is an epistemological shift – a shift in *a way of knowing* – between the first two sections of this book and the section that begins with radical empathy and moves through living compassion. The shift is simple but quite radical and transformative. Living compassion is a different way of knowing than "being compassionate" and radical empathy is a bridge meant to reveal living compassion for the subterranean common sense that it is.

The path is thus:

Threading the eye of the needle that is self-compassion leads to Step Two of this book, Compassion Toward Another. Radical empathy slides into the radiant truth of empathy and looks at the obstacles of self-involvement and "idiot compassion." This leads over the epistemological edge into the *mysterium* which this book is about ultimately: compassion is not ultimately an activity of the self but something vaster and incomprehensible. "Not I but God in me and through me." From the angle of living compassion one sees all the previous steps on the path as preparation to be a vehicle for this mystery. And indeed all the previous steps are quietly pervaded by the manifest and emergent reality of this mystery. "I" was never the Source of compassion.

Both empathy and living compassion depend first and foremost on presence, that pale, all too human reflection of Divine Presence or Light. It is into this light that suffering is received, ministered to. In some traditions this light itself is the presence of compassion.

17

Idiot Compassion

Straight out of nursing school, I spent four years at the bedside of Mildred cultivating a relationship with presence that has served me well in the rigors of hospital nursing where presence is so easily fragmented.

Mildred was a seventy-year-old Pentecostal woman with advanced multiple sclerosis. She'd been bedridden for thirty years, having only control over her facial muscles. A ventilator attached to a tracheotomy in her neck made it possible for her to breathe.

The routine was that I'd arrive at work at 11 p.m. We'd converse as well as we could for a half-hour, catching up, then I'd give her medications in applesauce and kiss her goodnight. Through the night I'd suction her occasionally and occasionally give her the bedpan. But mostly I learned about sitting still till the end of my shift. For four years I was a freelance monk.

Serious meditation practice means having a ringside seat at the circus of one's neuroses, aspirations, delusions, and a taste for melodramatic fantasy. One is merely watching the mind and the mind is a most curious creature. A lucidity emerges when one finally drops, exhausts, sees through, or simply laughs at this parade of illusions. At the heart of this raggedy practice is the cultivation of the present moment. With Mildred, the first layer of finding the presence was seeing past what the Vajrayana Buddhists call idiot compassion.

Idiot compassion feeds on the dualistic projection that I am the healthy, happy one and the recipient of my compassion is an afflicted, pitiable soul. Pity is a problem when one is feeling very noble about what a kind person one is. At its worst, it serves needs related to one's own self-image and functionally doesn't really see the human being inside of the pitied one.

For most of my first year with Mildred I got in touch with my inner idiot and to a measure took his opinions quite seriously. The way he saw it, Mildred was a variant of Christ crucified. Nailed to the cross or nailed to a diagnosis – what's the difference? Sooner or later I'd likely witness her death, wash her corpse. "Nursing duties." Images of the *pietá* would come. My spiritual practice those months, I thought, meant identifying with her evident anguish and hopefully thereby make a saint out of myself.

Mildred cured me of this delusion one night when I was feeling a little down. Arriving at work we soon stepped into our nightly conversation.

(One must understand Mildred couldn't talk because she was on a ventilator. I would read her lips inasmuch as it was possible and occasionally when both of us were nuts with frustration I'd take her off the vent for a few moments, squeeze an ambu bag into her trach and press enough air through her vocal cords for three or four well-chosen words. The simplest of conversations took a very long time.)

"How are you?" she asked.

"Oh, I'm a little sad."

"Why?"

"Life just seems sad to me sometimes."

"I rarely feel sad."

"How's that, Mildred? Some people would think you'd be pretty bitter about your life."

"I just don't let things bother me."

This was not a conversation with someone midway through her crucifixion. In a flash I saw that my earnest desire to be crucified alongside her was more than a little silly. This strange little fantasy collapsed to much laughter when I actually *saw* Mildred. I may have been dangling from my own cross back then, but Mildred most certainly wasn't. Mildred was a God-loving woman who was bathed in love. She didn't at all see her fate as tragic.

This amalgam of "saintliness" and narcissism says something about projections. In the theater of the soul, projection may think it's about another but it's actually about me-ness and that me was surely larger than life.

The withdrawal of projection allows the modest often invisible nature of compassionate activity. With Mildred it resolved sweetly to the warmth of our late nightly chats, protecting her sleep, turning her gently in bed, cleaning her when she soiled herself. And of course percussing her lungs, suctioning her, and giving her meds. All this embedded in long nights of learning to sit still.

Ego, projection and idiot compassion are of a piece. Likewise presence, seeing through and laughter.

In Buddhism the compassionate mind is a given (just as being created in God's image is a common understanding of the Judeo-Christian-Muslim tradition) Compassion (and being so created) is not to be achieved, it is in fact the natural order of things, what some teachers call "extraordinary ordinariness." With Mildred I came to appreciate the gentle rigorousness of this practice. The mind that is learning to sit still is pulled hither and thither by its desire to get spiritual, among other distractions. And yet things slowly begin to settle. "Before enlightenment, chop wood and carry water. After enlightenment, chop wood and carry water." With Mildred it was: before and after enlightenment, slide the bed pan under her bum, suction her, protect her sleep, and watch *The 700 Club* with her before reporting off to the oncoming shift.

Marty, a nurses aide, tells a similar story about dropping ego and projection.

Wake up! No nonsense. Samurai Zen. Fierce, direct, "sudden enlightenment."

Ivan was a twenty-two-year-old fellow in the Navy, stationed in San Diego. By the time he was admitted to the neurology floor, he was having a dozen epileptic fits a day. Marty's acquaintance with him lasted less than ten minutes.

At the beginning of the shift, Ivan's nurse, Karen, said to Marty, "Could you come down to 748? I need a big strong man." Feeling none too macho, he followed her.

Two other male personnel were trying to get restraints on Ivan. He was red-eyed, wild, spitting green sputum through his tracheotomy. ICU psychosis. Seizures were feeding a nervous breakdown, and the nervous breakdown was causing seizure activity. Karen needed him restrained so she could give him an Ativan injection into his thigh and break the cycle for awhile.

"For some reason, I wanted to look the beast in the eye," said Marty.

"I wanted. I! Too much 'I.' "

After we had his hands strapped to the bed, Marty looked straight into the fury of Ivan's eyes.

Ivan's response was precise. Like an archer flexing a bow and setting the arrow for the exact center, Ivan torqued his neck and then thrust his forehead toward the center of Marty's forehead.

Whack! End of a hallucination.

"I had made his torture a spectacle," said Marty.

My story of Mildred and Marty's story of Ivan bear the same teaching. Too much "I" distracts from the simple presence of living compassion. The recognition that Marty's "I" was making a spectacle out of his vast (idiot) compassion and the immediacy of Ivan's "thump," dislodged "I" and its melodramas.

Sasaki Roshi, the great Zen master now over a hundred years old, says, "I'm looking for the moment to throw you over the cliff." Ivan did just that. Marty saw his folly.

"Mentally, I thanked him," he said.

18

Narcissism Devours Presence

Narcissism is the most common variety of too much "I." Nothing distracts from the practice of compassion as effectively. Narcissism simply devours the possibility of the compassionate gesture.

On the door hung the name "Mrs. Akosian," but she most certainly was not Armenian. Mrs. Akosian was one of the great dancers of the twentieth century, and for twelve hours near the end of her life I was her nurse.

The silence of our time together lingers, and now, several years later, it poses essential questions about narcissism (and its bastard child, fandom) and the practice of radical empathy.

The heart of the story is very simple. Delighted that I was assigned Mrs. Akosian I made a point of entering her room with a bit of professional decorum.

Nonetheless, before meeting her, I quickly rehearsed the moment of checking her pedal pulses and saying, as if unrehearsed: "These are the feet of a great dancer!"

Was she going to be the young, sexy, radiantly American icon I knew from her fifties movies? I hadn't seen an image of her that was not this icon so I suppose there was a bit of reverence. And yet, the person lying in the bed was another woman altogether: watchful and silent, perhaps weary of hospital life. Paralyzed on her left side. Being called to death. Initial shock gave way to tender regard, but I couldn't waste the rehearsed moment. After taking vital signs and lung sounds, checking the placement of her IV and swabbing with betadine the pink stoma where her gastrointestinal tube entered her stomach, I peeled off her socks and smiled with "fresh spontaneity."

"These are the feet of a great dancer."

It was the right tone. Neither grave nor obtusely cheerful. No doubt a welcome break from the codes of an anonymous nurse and his supposedly anonymous patient. I was much pleased.

Mrs. Akosian listened silently. In fact, I don't recall any words being exchanged the whole night long.

In memory her silence persisted for years, until one night driving to work, something dislodged.

First the word "perhaps" began resonating.

Perhaps she was weary, the regimen of a long hospitalization, the revolving door of doctors and nurses poking and prodding at all hours of the day or night. Sometimes intimately. Sometimes painfully. The body belonging to everyone but herself.

Perhaps the grace of God came as anonymity. Many of her nurses were immigrants, others of a generation that would know nothing of her fame, and no doubt, some thought she was Mrs. Akosian.

Perhaps she was indifferent or perhaps flattered. When a cascade of "perhapses" engulfs a nurse on the way to work it doesn't take a wise one to point out the obvious: the beginning, middle, and end of this story is about me, or, more precisely, "me-ness" and its possible consequences.

Perhaps a public person at the end of her life doesn't need to be reminded of the woman she no longer is. She was now hemiplegic – hardly a dancer. Perhaps my praise of the great woman's feet was received as cruelty.

Contrary to the received wisdom, few of us will be famous for fifteen minutes, now or in the future. Many more, no doubt, are fated to the booby prize of, at least, a few moments of being a horse's ass before the silent presence of the famous. Mrs. Akosian's silence was perfect and pervasive. The cascade of "perhapses" and all its unanswerable questions left me with some of the essential Buddhist teachings about compassion.

In Vajrayana Buddhism, such narcissism, common as grass, is named the main obstacle to compassion. Lorne Ladner writes: "Tibetan Buddhist teachers note that for someone striving to develop compassion, self-cherishing is the principal inner enemy to be defeated. Hatred and anger are obvious enemies of compassion, but, in daily life, the simple tendency to cherish our self-image, comfort, security, possessions and status is the real enemy that chokes the very life of compassion."

"Yet, ordinarily," Ladner continues, "we don't notice our own narcissism, and our friends, family and culture support it." Years after my evening with Mrs. Akosian it came as a random thought that perhaps my contrived, self-conscious "spontaneity" had a blunt edge, unconscious in its hyper self-consciousness. Unconscious, that is, to her person.

Hospitals are hotbeds of narcissism, the pall over small interactions, the climate of perpetual complaint forever aggravated by understaffing. It's five-thirty in the morning and soon the shift will change. Finally, finally, things are starting to slow down, and damn if Mrs. Moore hasn't just died. Call the doc, the family, prepare the corpse, and take her to the morgue. Or there's an admit. Or Mr. Rodriguez is smeared with feces again. Or what's-his-name is confused and enraged.

We are all mortal and limited. And flawed. And there *is* great suffering in our efforts to minister to the suffering. But the culture of narcissism torques all this toward the strange fiction, the adamant hallucination, that it's our own suffering that truly matters in this ocean of suffering.

All of which is to say, my brief debut as Mrs. Akosian's registered horse's ass nurse was the "light side" of a cultural neurosis, both All-American but also universal.

All institutions and professions know their narcissistic style. What would it mean to do a study across professions of nurses, teachers, and prison guards? What the three share in common is that patient, student, and prisoner easily become the "other," sometimes even the enemy. The work life becomes embattled, the nurse's station a rampart against roiling chaos, the teacher's lounge or the circle of guards hunkered over black coffee – the same.

Do I exaggerate? Absolutely. Narcissism may be near the core of the human psyche, may be a cultural demon, forever sabotaging love with fictions of normality, but compassion is the deeper truth. Its possibility is always present.

Do I exaggerate?

Perhaps.

19

La Familia and Radical Empathy

Radical Empathy opens from a familiarity with oneself – with joy and sorrow – to meet another's.

Empathy is where two stories run parallel to each other and then meet.

It was one of those shifts on the oncology floor, the beginning of a double, and very busy. For the first three hours I did little but rush up and down the hall doing this or that. I kept passing a tough-looking Latino kid, maybe fifteen, weeping outside a patient's door. Couldn't possibly address whatever was happening with him – too much to do.

A couple of hours later it was a bit slower and there was much fuss around the nurse's station. It seems that Armando, that kid in the hall, had stuffed the public restroom sink with paper towels, turned on the water, and caused a little flood. The staff agreed to call security. "Just to scare him, that's all," said the secretary. More to the point, he and his extended family were gathered around his mother's bed. She was in the last stages of liver cancer and probably wouldn't last till morning.

I was called to act before security arrived, but I can't say I felt anything other than awkward and afraid. I had to consciously remember I'd seen a broken kid in the hall, a frightened child.

Courage is not about having no fear. It's when you honor the fear and act as you must.

Opening the door, I introduced myself. *La familia* listened expectantly while I talked clumsily in my mother's language to Armando.

"Armando, you flooded the bathroom, didn't you?"

He said "yes" weakly, his eyes to the side and down.

"When I was a few years older than you, my father died. I didn't know how to handle it at all. Is it true that you messed up the bathroom because seeing your mom like this made you feel too many things all at once?"

"Yes."

"And you're not a bad person and won't make any more trouble?"

"Yes."

"Take care of him," I said to his family. "His heart is breaking. Some of the staff got scared and called security. I'll send them away."

Empathy is located where two stories intersect. I was once a boy who lost a parent and, like Armando, confused in my grief, acted out. We shared the common knowledge of heartbreak. From that point where our stories connected I could respond not to the "bad boy," with humiliation or calls to security. The more compassionate way was sheltering the grief of a child who was seeing his mother die in front of him.

There was a flicker of grace in those few moments with Armando and his family. I knew I wouldn't see them again but we connected. I had prevented an act of violence born of ignorance, and Armando wouldn't forget it – just as I will never forget those who were kind to me when I was out of my mind with grief.

I'd walked many a moon in Armando's moccasins. Across the threshold I was able to see the moment of the dying of Armando's mother through his eyes and speak to him and his family accordingly.

The real stories are the stories that we live. Those are the true ones. The heart of the village lives in these stories. The Jewish philosopher Franz Rosenzwieg said the people look to scripture for parables that shed light on how they might live, but in reality the actual lived life is the source for parables that illuminate scripture. Doctors and nurses live such parables. From within the way of compassion, one lives out and scrutinizes a work that is true and meaningful. In this we begin to understand how .the spirit of kindness moves, for in any village, stories are the lifeblood.

Mike was twenty-three years old with metastatic brain cancer. A poor prognosis. His mind was slipping a little, and his deep concern was that his two-year-old daughter, the light of his life, would not remember him when he was gone.

Empathy for Mike came easily. I had a two-year-old daughter when I was his age and remembered well the sweetness of being a young man discovering what it is to be a father. My brief relationship with Mike was father to father, I to Thou, before it was nurse to patient.

Again the slide of radical empathy – seeing his life, his dying, and his little girl through his eyes.

For a couple of nights I helped him record the gist of what he wanted to convey to his child. Entering into Mike's story from the edge of my own, I helped craft the story of his life for Jessica so that the seed of who he was would be placed in her psyche. Mike finished by recording what it was to come to love Jessica while she swelled in her mother's belly, what it was to watch her be born at home, to cut her umbilical cord. What it was when she took her first steps, spoke her first words, when she saw the ocean for the first time and announced, "Milk!"

"Remember, little one, that though I am gone you were loved by your father. I give you now to your mother's arms."

It was a gift for Mike and a gift for me as well, reminding me of what is priceless. Here we see a little of the medicine of story, its many dimensions. Mike showed me clearly that the moment you meet a "Thou" you step into the story of common humanity, a textured, lived tale that included him and me and our daughters.

Common humanity is the only place where compassion can happen. That recognition is grace, sometimes redemption.

20

The Kindest of Buddhas

Armando's and Mike's stories are about radical empathy proceeding from deep familiarity. Jimmy's is about empathy in the wilderness of the unfamiliar.

To practice radical empathy in hell is to carry Buddha nature and in Japan, it is said that the kindest of Buddhas live in hell. In this chapter I want to pay homage to my teacher – which is to say, a patient who from behind eyes of terror taught me how to walk with presence in hell and how I might meet the spirit of kindness there.

Jimmy was thirty-five years old, homeless, psychotic, HIV positive, with a taste for liquor. Before he was admitted to UCLA Medical Center his life was undoubtedly hellish, but there are levels and levels of darkness and when I met Jimmy, it was as bleak as it gets. Quite drunk, he'd fallen asleep in the middle of the street in West L.A. and was run over by a car and was admitted with blood on the brain.

The surgery was successful enough, draining the hematoma, but after surgery he caught an infection in his cranial wound that was resisting antibiotics. Gowned up in a sterile paper gown, I donned a paper mask and carried the little plastic bottle of antibiotics into his isolation room where he was, in fact, isolated.

Having heard him from the hallway cursing and wailing I was aware that I was about to be with an intensely paranoid man and so I called on the spirit of kindness that I might somehow meet him in his torment. I found him tied down with wrist and ankle restraints and soaked in urine. And blood. He had pulled out his IV access and his skin was slick with HIV blood.

"We serve Christ in all his distressing disguises," said Mother Teresa. Jimmy was distressing all right and his distress amplified as I double-gloved to clean him. Lovely thoughts about kindness or Mother Teresa were now so much smoke in a windstorm. Soon Jimmy let me know I was the devil and screamed as I sponged him off.

Stick a needle in his vein, restart the IV? I left his room and called the doctor to change the antibiotic order to a pill. Trying to compose myself the question begged to be answered: What could kindness possibly mean, what is its essential activity, its sacred gesture, when one has inarguably become the devil in a man's private hell?

Reentering Jimmy's room and putting on the persona of a professional nurse I handed him the pill. His response was that of any sensible madman offered poison by the devil – he spat in my face and shouted, "Get out of here, Satan."

Leaving the room again, hell now spread in ten directions. Jimmy's future looked as bitter as his present – get the infection under control and transfer him to a psych facility, which would likely transfer him eventually back to the street. Knowing that it is not possible to ignore a treatable brain infection, I conscripted Maria, an ICU nurse known for her deft fingers, to start the necessary IV.

Holding firmly his wrist while a nurse's aide pinned his shoulder, his fury mounted as Maria tied latex around the biceps and looked for a vein. Lost and heartbroken over the tragic impossibility of it all, I closed my eyes knowing that momentarily the needle would pierce his flesh.

Nurses, like other professionals who week by week return to hell, often place such moments in "parentheses" or into tidy boxes in their minds that aren't at all true to the ragged untidiness of what we do. Who can bear the raw truth of it day after day? With Jimmy, I chose not to make the situation other than it was, to be simply present before rage and anguish. His bloodcurdling screams washed over me, and for a few moments it seemed they preceded right from the heart of God.

At 3 a.m. it was time for my hour of meditation. I decided to spend it in his room. Jimmy was sound asleep and I sat across from him and practiced *tonglen*, the Tibetan practice of inhaling another's suffering and exhaling loving kindness. In Buddhist practice one meditates with one's eyes open and so in this intimate hour I was able to settle into the beauty of the man on the other side of his masque of torment.

Tonglen dissolves the territoriality of ego, undoes the defended heart. Compassion is realized - or remembered - in giving it away. The nun Pema Chodron describes the process of *tonglen* thus:

"First, rest your mind briefly, for a second or two, in a state of openness or stillness.

"Second, work with texture. Breathe in a feeling of hot, dark and heavy - a sense of claustrophobia - and breathe out a feeling of cool, bright and light - a sense of freshness."

The extremity of anguish insists on spiritual questions perhaps unanswerable, or at least not to be answered superficially. What is the nature of this life that some are born to this or fated to stagger into it? And why he and not I? Surely God suffers the fact of it, perhaps participates in the truth of it and perhaps that participation is the fount of Divine compassion. I could not in any way diminish Jimmy's suffering, but I could find the courage to bear witness to it.

I call Jimmy a teacher because washing his bloody body and having his screams washing me deepened my faith in the spirit of kindness. Walking on the beach with my wife a couple of evenings later my legs gave way as I told the story. Jimmy cleansed me of a whole world of delusion about the path of compassion. Once an earnest young Catholic given to believing the generosity of his goodness would diminish the vastness of suffering itself, I was laughing now at the presumptuousness and threw a stone into the waves. "Like pebbles to the sea, trying to fill it up," I said. Jimmy taught that the way of compassion is far more real, more honest and humble, genuinely generous.

One cannot take personally the spit and foul language of a man who is quite over the edge. One doesn't choose who deserves and doesn't deserve kindness. What is tragic or even unimaginably hopeless calls for the spirit of kindness, and so the heart must remain open in hell. No act of kindness is misbegotten, even if it's merely being present and bearing witness. Undistracted by futility and thus undistracted by concerns of being effective, the momentary willingness to be undefended allowed the spirit of kindness to instruct in the most uncompromising way. His darkness and terror stripped me of the naiveté and personae that cramp and falsify the compassionate gesture.

21

Surviving Something No One Should Survive

Ana was a nurse who for years I knew only when I'd report off to her at the end of night shift or she to me at the end of her day shift. It was in report that she was told of a patient that she had when she was a young nurse in Miami. We got together for breakfast later in the week and she filled out the story of Ramona.

Ramona, a lawyer for Amnesty International, was for twelve years tortured in a small South American country.

Ana's story perfectly illustrates radical empathy and clarity that was the edge of compassion in an extraordinary situation.

Ramona had tried to commit suicide by not eating, just as she had tried in prison. She had been found by one of her friends, who called 911.

"She was so weak she couldn't stand and was causing 'problems' – screaming at people and not allowing them to do anything. She ripped out her IV so she couldn't be fed with peripheral nutrition."

Ramona had been force-fed in prison and was outraged that now that she was free, the prison of the hospital would tether her to an IV and force-feed her.

"Even before I came to her room I was told, 'you have to come. There's a big problem going on right now.' "

"The nurse's aide was standing over her with her arms crossed like a bear and Ramona was almost pleading. I recognized this woman had been tortured and was not herself."

When Ana told me this story what I noticed was a pivoting of her psyche. She could see the nurse's aide trying to be tough through the eyes of a woman who had suffered years of torture.

" 'Who are you? Are you like her?' she asked me."

"No, I'm not her. My name is Ana and I'm your nurse and I'm going to make sure she doesn't come in your room again."

Ana works with horses, and she recognized in this woman a wounded animal. "When a horse is wounded you grab her and get very physical. I completely went into feeling her need and I sat next to her and put my arm around her. She just dissolved into sobbing and started telling me these horrible, horrible visions of how her family was murdered in front of her."

Because of Ramona's work with human rights she had been imprisoned as an enemy of the state. She had been raped upwards of a thousand times and now had cervical cancer.

"For over an hour I held her like a baby and she sobbed and sobbed. Of course I had other patients, but the charge nurse was sensitive to what we were in. She assigned my patients to other nurses so I could follow through with Ramona. She protected my space so I could protect Ramona's space."

"Doctors came and went. They sat, asked a few questions. Most of the doctors were very understanding. When they saw what was going on, they left. I barely looked at them. I continued my absolute, one hundred percent complete body-soul focus on Ramona and her need at that moment."

After her initial outburst Ramona confessed that what she really wanted was a cigarette. Ramona was on suicide prevention so she was not to leave the unit to smoke. Nonetheless Ana said, "I will make sure you get a cigarette."

The hospital was able to reassign an aide who would sit with Ramona, and Ana introduced her.

"Is she going to be like the last one?"

"I'll make sure she's not like the last one."

"Is it okay if we walk out of the room and I tell her your story so she can understand what you need?"

Ana was quite aware that she was speaking to Ramona like this in front of the aide and could feel the aide's resistance in the air. In the hallway Ana told the aide that Ramona had seen her family shot in front of her and had been tortured and raped for defending the tortured.

"I just appealed to her. She became another person, completely transformed from 'what are you going to tell me I have to do today that I don't want to do today' to 'man, I'm right here with you; I'll do anything you want me to do with her.' "

And she had a cigarette!

"That, my dear, is your ticket to this woman right now."

She completely softened to the task of saving the victim, and when they returned to the room Ana said, "She is meant to be here with you! She even has a cigarette, so let's go."

Unconcerned with the rules of suicide watch, Ana helped Ramona into a wheelchair, and the aide took her to a fire escape to enjoy smoking.

"A whole herd of doctors came. 'Where is she? What have you done with her?'"

"She's having a cigarette."

"What, are you ...!" And I said, "Sometimes the most important thing in the world is a cigarette!"

Ana is not a smoker.

"I'll take you to where she is. She's on the fire escape with the aide that's watching her. She's completely compliant."

The doctors were quite angry with Ana's crazy talk about a cigarette and about letting Ramona out of her room. Undaunted, when the doctors reached the fire escape door, Ana insisted on conferring with Ramona before letting the doctors see her.

"Your doctors are behind the door. They want to see you. Do you want to see them?"

"I asked her permission every step of the way. She said, 'I'll talk to one of the doctors.'"

Ana, again, was seeing the institution of the hospital through the eyes of a woman who knew the institution of prison. Initially Ramona had said, "I am a lawyer. I know my rights, and I decide whether I eat or not." But at the end of the day she was eating. And she was even beginning to stand on her own.

"She was so emaciated, she was a hollow skeleton. I could pick up her body in my arms, and she was not that small. When I saw her trying to stand, my first impulse as a nurse was to stop her because I didn't want her to fall. I walked over and put my arm around her."

"I was in a real moral dilemma with Ramona. Because I found myself communicating with her in her dire pain I was able to speak directly, and I told her she had been condemned to bear witness. No one was supposed to survive something like this. We talked of Elie Wiesel meeting his friend's eyes at Auschwitz as he was being executed. Like Wiesel, she was condemned to bear witness to the suffering of the tortured."

Ana knew she was totally outside her bounds as a nurse. "What right did I have to tell this woman anything like that? Where did I get off insisting that she live?"

It was then Ramona told her the story that broke her.

"They injected me so I had no free use of my limbs and then they lifted my hand and forced me to shoot my son."

"She was holding her hand out like it was not part of her body and said, 'This hand, this hand killed my boy.' "

Ana took her hand and put it to her face and said, "This hand did not belong to you. This hand was not your hand. They used your trigger finger to kill your boy and break you. *They* shot your son, not you."

Ana told me she didn't know where this came from.

"Who am I to challenge that kind of pain? What is my right? I asked her how many people she had told this to."

"Three. I was the third."

"Of course you want to die," said Ana. "And you have every right to die."

Ana could see that Ramona was at the crossroads, choosing life or death, and she empathized with either choice. Speaking of Elie Wiesel was a way of reframing why in fact she might choose to live. Receiving the story of how her torturers appropriated her hands to kill her son left Ana no argument with why she would want to exit this life. Ana gave credence to both options as she offered Ramona coffee, eight creamers, and lots of sugar. She wanted Ramona to live, but she protected the woman's integrity of choice moment to moment.

"She was looking out the window and I knew she was back in prison because she was staring at the brick wall of the next building. I said, 'You want to see something really beautiful? Follow me.' We took the elevator to the eighth floor and watched the doves, iridescent, on the rooftops below. It all boiled down to moving from prison to life."

Ana stepped into the ethical complexity of the elder, rich in ambiguity.

By empathically sliding into Ramona's mind, Ana's allegiance for Ramona's autonomy became the blade of discernment for Ana herself.

With this discernment Ana was able to make choices wisely in the moment. If Ana had conceded to the way a hospital routinely compromises a patient's autonomy, she would simply have been recognized as one more among Ramona's torturers.

Ana stayed in touch with Ramona for a while after she was released from the hospital. The last she heard, Ramona was spending her mornings and early afternoons trying to get political prisoners released in South America, and also in the Middle East. This gave her life meaning; occasionally her efforts as a lawyer were successful. The rest of the day and into the evening she returned to the questions of continuing to live or choosing not to.

Step Four

Living Compassion

About Living Compassion

It is said in heaven there is no scarcity. Nourishment is abundant yet we feed each other. In hell the illusion of scarcity torments and we eat greedily from our plates and other's too.

From the *mysterium* of living compassion I invite you to heaven.

No self and no other is how Glaser explains the *mysterium*, the (non)vision that is *living compassion*. I will try to describe it, though the lived truth is outside of language. Glaser merely says, "The self-other axis *cannot* be separated from the no-self – no-other axis if our compassion is to achieve full expression. Both are equally true, but taken alone, each is false. Self and other, and no-self and no-other, must be understood as co-existing and interdependent realities if we hope to find the grail of compassion."

Just as self-compassion done for real *slips* into compassion for others, *radical empathy* can give way into the spaciousness and clarity of *living compassion*.

"To study Zen is to study the self. To study the self is to forget the self. To forget the self is to be enlightened by all things," says Dogen Zenji.

Across cultures *living compassion* reverberates from "not I but Christ in me," and the Muslim *fatiya* of forgetting oneself in God's will. I and Thou momentarily drops away and one is amidst the forever plural truth of living beings, loving them unconditionally.

Unconditional love is another way of expressing *living compassion*.

In this, one is enlightened by all things.

You are no longer self-consciously kind towards another –
you step forth *as* compassion, un-self-consciously. You are fully
identified with the process of compassionate activity.

You know when you have entered into *living compassion*
when the profound gift nature of the loving act reveals itself. You
are not living compassion if you are expecting anything in return.

Living compassion is the essential nature of human freedom.

And *living compassion* is pure gift. Zadie Smith describes it
precisely:

"The moment when the ego disappears and you're able to
offer up your love as a gift without expectation of reward. At this
moment the gift hangs, between the one who sends and the one
who receives, and reveals itself as belonging to neither."

Compassion as a presence – as *Presence* – is most relevant
here. The person who meets this or that situation compassionately
is vehicle for this quality that the bottom line of which is not
personal. The spiritual practice of *living compassion* requires that the
self step aside. It is radically and blessedly simple, and its
experience extraordinarily ordinary. Compassion is the
environment that one is in. One is alert to its presence, available
to being its vehicle but one doesn't for a moment *possess*
compassion.

22

Kindness Is a Spirit

When I met Lewis I was not well. I'd just returned from Africa and my body and soul were in the African time of my friends – which is to say a slowness not at all compatible with what is required to make it from one end of a twelve-hour shift to another. I took to the poison, of course – half a dozen cups of coffee – thinking it would help me meet the tasks at hand. No go. I was in a dream, agitated, the other staff members spinning around me like so many drunken dervishes. And so when I was told at 3 a.m. that I had an admit, I was less than enthused. Nonetheless, when I came to the door of his room I took a deep breath and sighed a hopeless, exhausted prayer, "Make use of me."

Lewis was fifty-five years old, Down syndrome, his head a lopsided melon bulging in front, his hands and feet curled up, a wheelchair at his bedside because he couldn't walk. His elderly mother had brought him to the hospital because he had a nasty infected abscess in his left foot.

Admitting Lewis, I got a little of his story - very little, very sparse. His father had died recently and it was not altogether clear how long his mother would live. And then? An institution, I suppose, but it wasn't the content of his story that touched me so much as his inscrutable manner. The lack of self-pity or melodrama could certainly be read as a cognitive deficit, but the inscrutable nature of our interaction left me stranded between interpretations.

An imbecile? A holy one? Neither or both? I simply could not read him.

"You are a remarkable man," I told him later as I cleaned his wound, laid strips of wet saline gauze across it, and wrapped it in Kerlix dressing.

"Thank you," he replied.

Did he understand what I meant? I left his room feeling put back together again, grateful and humbled by a humble soul.

Where was the spirit of kindness with Lewis? In him? In me? Or hovering between us in the neon glare as he told of his father's death while I tended his wound? It was my meeting with Lewis that convinced me that the spirit of kindness is indeed a spirit, for I could not locate it but was nonetheless healed by it. The closest I can get is to say that the meeting itself healed me of my fragmentation. Lewis's story carries light, gentle, and lucid, and through the simplicity of two men meeting across worlds I learned that compassionate activity itself is medicine. I was incoherent before we met, and was rendered whole. I could not find the thread until we received one another.

Lewis drew something out of me that was new and unanticipated, and I've tried to fold the lessons into the day-to-day life of living compassion inside and outside the hospital. To approach each patient's room, each interaction, with quietly stated intent, hopeful, hopeless but reaching towards being available to kindness. Yes - to keep the faith with the intent. And then we meet - I to Thou. Stark as he was, in The Kindest of Buddhas chapter, Jimmy taught me the most essential lesson - the most essential - that the spirit of kindness arrives when one dares to bear witness. It all begins with simple presence, the simple willingness to say "this one is a human being like myself." Without this, there is no meeting. Without meeting, there is no compassion. Without compassion, the hands and heart are numb and there will be no living gesture of touching another.

In a modern hospital the spirit of kindness "bloweth where it listeth." One can be responsive to its presence but cannot control it. One can only be hospitable to it, alert to its movement in oneself, one's coworkers, or patients in whatever situation.

And one can be attentive to the crazy discipline of being available as its vehicle. This is a fierce and glorious path. Fortunately, there are many teachers and, as they say, "a teacher touches infinity." It is for us to recognize them, discern their teachings, and live by what we learn.

With Lewis, the self-other axis was illuminated by a third – the spirit of kindness – and with that there was an aware self-forgetting. The thought of *me* being compassionate toward *him* would be simply false. He and I met in the *environment* of compassion, radiant and fresh.

My time with Lewis adds a twist of paradox to Shakespeare:

> *The quality of mercy is not strained.*
> *It droppeth as the gentle rain from heaven*
> *Upon the place beneath, it is twice bless'd*
> *It blesses him that gives and him that takes.*

Lewis and I were thrice blessed because the spirit of kindness allowed us for a few moments to extend and receive mercy from each other.

Self and other – I and Thou – are not abolished by no-self, no-other. They are contained within this selflessness but they also lend body and ground to selflessness. They are necessary to one another, interdependent truths.

The sacred nature of plurality is honored as is the meeting of two that gives birth to an angel.

23

Love Is the Only Medicine I Know

The gift nature of compassionate activity was made vividly clear a few years ago. I'd come to work early and spent a couple of hours meditating and praying in the hospital chapel. Before I left to the neuro floor for a twelve-hour shift, I'd settled into that relaxed, open lucidity that sometimes comes with sitting still. I began my shift as ready as I'd ever been to face the challenges with poise and generosity.

Or so I thought.

I had too many patients, all but one of them confused and agitated: Mr. Owen (the unconfused one), an aging hippie eager to regale me with stories of the olden days; Mrs. Suarez, out of her skin with Alzheimer's and trying to get out of her bed with a broken hip; Mr. Cohen, delusional with alcohol withdrawal; and young Billy, jonesing for methamphetamines.

All of these were "manageable," requiring mere damage control. And then there was Carmen.

Carmen was in her early twenties, had been afflicted with seizure activity from the time she was a child, and with this admission was having several fits a day. She was practically feral in her demeanor, tied to her bed with an impatient nurse's aide at her bedside to ensure she didn't harm herself. She'd spit at you, her aim true, bite you if you weren't careful, would no doubt scratch your eyes out if her hands weren't tied down. Hell has a center where pain reaches an extreme pitch. Carmen was strapped to that place.

I was obviously flailing. The floor was busy, but my workload was beyond the pale. Living compassion rose up on behalf of me - and through me, on behalf of Carmen. A nurse here and an aide there stepped forth to check one of my patient's blood sugar, to do another's vital signs, to draw blood for another, to check medication records against recent doctor's orders. These small gestures made it possible for me to extract myself from the shift's cascade of little crises and approach Carmen's bedside with a modest measure of balance and tenderness – and to extend support to her aide, who was agitated and impatient sitting alongside the volatility of Carmen's suffering hour after hour. I did the ordinary nursing tasks – checking her vital signs, emptying her Foley catheter of urine, giving her morning medications with apple sauce (which she'd spit back at me), and singing to her in Spanish while I did so. (Carmen was from Guatemala.)

At 3 a.m. I took refuge in a shower closet to spend an hour meditating. It took perhaps forty minutes to simply steady my breath. Eventually something profound dawned on me, so obvious yet I'd been blind to it.

Yes, it was about this shift, but more broadly, it was about the nature of compassion.

It is an ordinary kind of egotism to imagine that I am the source of the compassion I am able to give. Compassion is not something anyone possesses. It is a gift that I was being given that I might extend it to another.

Self-compassion, being the object of kindness and extending kindness became the indivisible whole they always were.

Every gesture of compassion has a village behind it – from the uncle who first saw the light that is in you when you were child and let you know it, to the nurse who, seeing your overwhelm, took a couple of sets of vital signs and freed you up to tend to a patient's anguish. Congratulating myself that I could be so relentlessly kind is so utterly beside the point. Gratitude and humility within the general conspiracy *is* the point.

I scribbled the poem:

> Love is the only medicine
> I know
> And I know it is not mine
> Passed swift from Lover to Beloved
> Woven from hand to hand

the gift given
never owned
utterly ordinary and also, perhaps
A song
to God that is love itself
who knows what healing is
as I most certainly do not

24

Without Thinking about Compassion, It Flows

Conversation with Jalaledin Ebrahim

Raised in Kenya, East Africa, educated in Paris and at Cornell University, Jalaledin Ebrahim is, like his spiritual master, His Highness the Agha Khan, a planetary citizen. Ultimately he studied spiritual psychology at the University of Santa Monica in California and got a second degree in counseling psychology from the Institute of Transpersonal Psychology in Palo Alto, California. He now works two nights a week in a psychiatric facility as well as full time as wrap-around facilitator with kids and families at risk. For him Islam is about surrender and service, two faces of one life in the Spirit. Here are his reflections on compassionate activity.

Michael: You work with those who are most marginalized by the culture: the mad and the emotionally disturbed. What is your approach?

Jalaledin: I had just graduated from the University of Santa Monica in spiritual psychology when I applied for this wrap-around position. In my job interview I was given a vignette. I was asked what would my answer be if I had this troubled kid under my care who was doing such and such. Because of my training I came to understand that each individual has their own answer so I said, "I don't have the answer. The child has the answer."

This is the essence of compassion. A person is a spiritual being with a human experience and the most I can do is support them in seeking their own answer. There is no sense of "fixing" people.

I was hired on the spot. I knew I was home because the director and I had a common language.

In this job we work with the strengths of the individual. We don't work with pathology. Instead of focusing on the illness, we empower people in their wellness. The illness dissipates on its own and wellness comes to the fore. It's an awesome thing to watch unfold.

Michael: Could you give me an example about how you apply that concretely?

Jalaledin: I worked with a seventeen-year-old guy who was in a shelter for a year and a half. His mother was a vagrant and his father was nowhere to be found. The social worker couldn't find him a foster home. Our team tried all sorts of things to no effect, so I decided to just let go and took him for a joy ride through the community just to get him out of the shelter where he was forever surrounded by these institutional symbols. We were driving into the Santa Cruz Mountains and were passing the Walden West Outdoor Science School when he said, "I've been here before! I was here when I was in sixth grade!"

I asked, "Do you want to go in and look around?"

He said, "Sure," and so we did.

Something happened. He was really excited to be there. I asked, "Would you like to volunteer here if I could find a place for you?"

He spent five nights as cabin supervisor with fifth and sixth graders, responsible for getting them up in the morning, taking them on hikes, being part of the team. I picked him up on the sixth day and he was completely different. He said he had these rave reviews by his supervisors and they'd invited him back anytime.

I actually didn't trust his story so I dropped him off at the shelter and called the program director and he said that his boy was amazing. The kids loved him! The staff loved him. Everyone loved him.

The program drew on his strengths and creativity and this dissipated the confusion of the previous year and half in the shelter. He became the healer. He had to care for these kids. He was recognized for his possibilities and stepped into them.

Michael: That's a profound statement. Not to be distracted by pathology but to move from a recognition of possibility instead.

Jalaledin: Exactly. In a psych facility you have to move from compassion and empathy because it's impossible to understand rationally how the patients see themselves or the universe.

Occasionally I find myself frustrated because something is outside of my paradigm of understanding. I can get frustrated or upset or angry. I was working with a woman in a manic episode. She was having an especially difficult night: unable to sleep, racing thoughts. Basically she didn't want me in her space. She said she saw me with an erection and if I didn't behave myself she would talk to an attorney. None of this made sense but I got caught up in her story and got really upset. She taught me how easy it is to lose center when you're being attacked by someone you're trying to support.

I started to read Edward Padvoll's book, *Recovering Sanity*. He writes about how easy it is to be seduced by another person's madness. I realized I had become "mad" in the sense that I'd entered into the madness of my client.

All of us have our moments of complete insanity. Once you recognize your own insanity you can become more compassionate with people who are suffering mental illness. Until you realize your own insanity you can't be fully compassionate. The mad one reveals to you your own vulnerability.

This work has been a huge blessing to me. I can't presume anyone is in the same place psychologically, emotionally or spiritually as I am. I am constantly required to relate to the individual nature of wherever a person's soul might be.

Michael: So this woman was your teacher, pushing the envelope, as it were, in learning compassion.

Jalaledin: When I was getting my training at the Institute of Transpersonal Psychology, we learned Aikido not as a martial art but as a way of meeting the energy the "opponent" brings towards you. You turn with the opponent and the energy of conflict dissipates. You come alongside them and support their energy wherever it is going. Basically, you get out of the way.

That attitude works well with the chronically mentally ill. Eventually I learned how to do that with this manic woman.

Michael: How does your practice as a Muslim inform what you do?

Jalaledin: Completely! I am a *Shia imami ismaili* Muslim, a follower of His Highness Agha Khan, who is a direct descendent of the prophet Mohammed, may peace be upon him. He is a very progressive planetary citizen. Ramadan is a holy month but fasting is not restricted to food and water. Fasting is a 365-days-a-year spiritual discipline. In this practice I pray for all living beings. On Thursday and Friday nights I leave the prayers to go to work at 10 p.m., so I'm in this amazing space of clarity and peace. My job is to make sure the house is peaceful at night.

My practice definitely affects my work. Without thinking of compassion it flows on its own. It's not a conscious thing. It just seems to be there. The concept of service is very important. My practice has two faces: surrender and service to the world. You cannot love Allah without loving his creation. The best way to express that love is to serve my fellow beings.

At the same time, it is so necessary to find replenishment when you work with such suffering. I spend a lot of time in nature. I have a massage every week. I pray and I meditate. Replenishment itself is a spiritual practice.

In my personal practice Jesus is always present. He is very important to Muslim people. On my altar I have a photograph of Agha Khan and the Dalai Lama and a picture of Jesus in a cloak of many colors. In Islam we speak of God as "Most Compassionate, Most Merciful." We speak of *baraka*, the spiritual abundance that comes through all of us. It's the experience of grace, blessing, and abundance.

The bigotry towards Islam is like all bigotry. It's always based on simple ignorance. All of us are so ignorant of other people, of other cultures. Suffering comes from ignorance. Mohammad's teaching was about overcoming ignorance.

25

Awakening to Who You Have Become

A vibrant community must have elders. The community of those who tend to the ill is no exception.

These elders are the ones who have been seasoned by suffering and what it is to work with the raw truth of it. They are the ones who have transformed a measure of their suffering to the compassionate gesture.

They are the ones who step forth.

For many it's been the facing of extremity that has tempered us and awakened us to possibility.

Dr. Karen Mutter tells her ordeal of "waking up" to what she routinely did as an intern in a hospital in New Jersey: "When I look back at myself in medical school, I realize I was asleep to what I was doing much of the time. But there were particular moments when I woke up, and they were excruciatingly painful. One particular time, I had been working in an ICU, had been awake thirty hours, and I was the first responder to resuscitate a ninety-year-old man, skin and bones."

"In a few moments everyone was there – the respiratory tech and the other residents. I jumped in and started pumping on his chest, hearing his ribs cracking. It was then that the veil lifted. I woke up and looked upon this dead man. I gave the code to another resident and left the ICU.

"I went back to my apartment and cried for hours. I was really scared. I thought I was losing my mind.

"I called a resident who lived down the hall. She was a couple of years ahead of me and carried a maturity I relied on. I told her I'd been crying for hours and I couldn't stop.

"She did the most brilliant thing. She took me to the park. All I could see and hear was this old man's face and the cracking of his ribs. It was so unnatural, and at the same time the park was radiant with spring, everything new. She was able to convey that there is a right order to everything and that I would be okay."

"Waking up" within her sleepless exhaustion to find herself cracking the rib cage of an old man is a waking up to the excruciating truth of what we do sometimes in the name of medicine. But the "older sister" quietly led Karen to another awakening – nature at its most alive restoring her. Keeping faith with the natural world is one way that makes the rigor of our work possible.

It is said that a woman whose daughter had died came to the Buddha to plead that he raise her from the dead. "I will do so," said the Buddha, "but first you must bring me a mustard seed from a house where no one has suffered the loss of a loved one."

Loss is a common truth, but there is a threshold one must cross to know this.

The elder does not indulge the fantasy of the uniqueness of his or her suffering or imagine it is others that suffer, not oneself. To know sympathetic sorrow requires looking without naïveté at the substance of what it is to be human. And any joy that seeks to be innocent of sorrow is a superficial thing, utterly unconvincing.

Ann Jyoshi is not one to shrink from the forthrightness sometimes required by an elder, including defending the dignity of the dead. "He was eighty years old, not even my patient. His nurse, Joan, a friend of mine, told me he so much wanted to die and kept pulling off his oxygen. So they restrained his wrists."

"She had had a long conversation with him during the day. They had an extraordinary rapport. He was lucid, not desperate, entirely sane. 'It's time for me to go,' he said. 'All I have to do is to take off this damn oxygen mask.'"

She told him she was going to go on a long break as she untied his restraints.

Together she and Ann went outside, lying on the grass beneath the ecstasy of the stars.

"I remember that night clearly. It was absolutely gorgeous. She told me about him under the crispness of a winter night in Albuquerque. We knew he was likely dying as we talked."

When they came back to the floor, much present in the mystery of the moment, they were disturbed to hear giggling behind the patients closed door. Ann recognized the voices – a nurse and a nurse's aide.

"Even before I opened the door something passed through me. I knew he was dead and the giggling of these girls – I call them 'girls' because of their immaturity – did not bode well. Before I opened the door I knew that I would have to bear witness to an outrage."

When Joan and Ann went into the patient's room they found him dead, propped up with reading glasses and his hands holding a newspaper.

Ann knew she had to defend his spirit. "I knew I had a job that I had to do. I'm not one who speaks up easily and I'm not a religious person or someone who believes in the occult, but this made a doubter into a believer.

"Joan and I told the girls 'get out. You have done something terrible. Get out.' I felt his presence in the room, not this cartoon they had made of his body. I felt he appointed me to speak up."

Sarah Deering's moment of awakening came after a string of personal deaths. She was at work when it was her mom's turn. Her story is telling and touching because it emblematized the moment she received the torch of eldership from her mother.

These past few years of Sarah's seasoning as a nurse in a small community hospital in Watsonville, California had been thick with one death after another – her father, a couple of dear friends, an old lover she had lived with for a few years.

And now her mom.

It was near the end of a long shift when Sarah picked up a long-distance call from the ambulance crew that was attempting to revive her mother. Her brother felt it would be best if she could be in touch at this moment, as the emergency technicians needed to know when it might be time to give up and let her mother pass. Minute by minute, moment by moment, she was apprised of what was happening hundreds of miles away. The cardiac rhythms. The oxygen saturation of her blood. And then – the end.

Rousing herself she hung up the phone. She knew it was right for her to complete her shift. "That's what my mother would want me to do."

A couple of months later Sarah worked alongside a student nurse. All day long trying to keep alive an elderly patient, repeatedly trying to strike the balance between insulin and blood sugar level. When the patient died she and the student went into the hallway, held each other and cried. "She was self-conscious about her tears," Sarah said. "I told her to never lose that. Always keep the edge between compassion and getting the job done."

26

The Presence of the Everyday

Conversation with Katherine Brown-Saltzman, RN

Katherine Brown-Saltzman has been a nurse for thirty years, almost all of that spent in pediatric and adult oncology, hospice, and palliative care. She was also briefly a teacher of preschool, poverty level. "That was my respite. I came back to oncology." She has taught me much about the craft of compassion. A picture of warmth and grace, our brief conversations in the hallways of UCLA Medical Center were refreshing. In the midst of the wild necessity of doing this or that, I was always aware of the unspoken – she a co-conspirator in the activity of kindness. And so there was deep pleasure in listening to her speak so freely about what is dear to our hearts: how the spiritual life informs caring for the ill.

Michael: I've observed you these years with a lot of respect and affection. You carry light in the hospital. How did you come to so value the work of compassion?

Katherine: I can't imagine doing this work without compassion. I remember as a child holding that place of compassion, seeing that there was pain and suffering I didn't understand. I was gifted with an openness to that and no need to run away from it. As I made the choice to work with the dying, this unfolded more. In this work you must figure out how to keep your heart open, literally broken open. When I'm with suffering, I ask, "What am I doing here?" and then, "How can I be helpful?"

I babysat in a large family when I was an adolescent and one of the children was diagnosed with leukemia. From there I went into nursing school, and while I trained I watched what that family went through and ultimately that child's death. That shifted me into thinking about childhood and death, what families needed, what was missing. In my senior year in college I did an independent study of death and dying, focusing on children.

Michael: Your true education in compassion required a lot of heartbreak. A child's death is especially hard.

Katherine: Yes, and during that summer I had another pivotal experience of working as a nurse's aide at night among dying patients. They were at the end of the hall; the door closed, abandoned, in terrible pain – physically, emotionally, spiritually. I was a nineteen-year-old kid, but somehow I had the ability to be present, to hear their stories and not be frightened. I could see not only the impact I had on them for not running away but theirs on me as well. Those were pivotal moments.

And then there are your own losses and you get broken in a different way. Having the heart broken again and again has been the way I've learned openness and compassion. Pretty simple.

I grew up in a very traditional, religious, Catholic family. This background filled with ritual and spiritual reading also opened a door for me in terms of having something to tap into. When this pivotal moment happened, I had this spiritual foundation to back me up.

There is heart and spirit but there's also the element of the mind. As nurses, we are constantly assessing. Part of that is intuition and part of it is the mind, keen to take things in and piece things together. I think compassion for the most part comes from heart and spirit.

The problem with the mind is that it sometimes gets in the way because the mind constantly judges. It tries to assert certain value on suffering: "This is so terrible, this is so terrible!" instead of returning to the heart and saying: "This is. How can I be present for this person?"

Michael: How do you make sense of such suffering without judging it?

Katherine: Suffering is a given I don't pretend to understand. It can be transformative. Over and over I've seen it shift people into making decisions about their life, their values. Yes, suffering can strike people down like lightning, but most of the time it doesn't. More often, it's transformative for people and transformative for those around them. When I behold suffering, it's not as if I'm not taken aback by it and wounded by it sometimes. But now, after thirty years, I don't merely observe suffering. I can be present to it, I can touch it, I can hold it. I can even, to a certain extent, try and heal it. What I used to do is just suck it in, and there it festered and made me useless.

Now I bear witness. There is a wonderful balance of being present to it and not letting it enter in a way that destroys you.

There is the collective suffering. Every time you bear witness to suffering, be it a patient, a family member, staff, the world, you are imprinted. I think it's like a glass window with the fingerprints of at first just a few people, then more and more, till pretty soon you have difficulty seeing. That's what I mean by the collective. Every time you come into a hospital you are imprinted. You get on an elevator and you see the ache in people's bodies and in their eyes. So you have to, on a regular basis, do a cleansing.

Michael: A cleansing?

Katherine: For myself, it's important for me to take a walk, take in the beauty of the world. Take in the feel of the ground, not walking on cement. Connecting. Prayer. Meditation. Gardening. Pruning. Planting.

The work that I do with patients can be meditation. I lay my hands on them and go into meditative states, layer after layer getting out of the way. To be as completely as possible there but not there. Being in meditative states for part of my work every day has saved me.

Michael: Prayer and meditation, then, are an intrinsic part of your day to day work.

Katherine: I try to pray every morning and throughout the day. When I walk into a patient's room, I will pray. When I make a phone call, I will pause and pray first.

When I used to do hospice home care in the East, where there were miles between patients, I had much time to pray as I drove. When I came here, it was just one door to another, and I really had to be conscious of not losing that precious time to drop away, to let go, to un-hinder, to get ready for pushing open that next door. It was really a challenge to condense what had happened during a beautiful ten- or twenty-minute drive into moments.

Not easy.

The frenetic activity level of the hospital and the tightness of the space do not encourage this kind of emotional availability. How do I, in the midst of the chaos, find the thread of awareness? It takes a concerted effort, but it's well worth it even if it's met only in a moment through deep breathing or taking one's self out of the chaos for a bit. It's so essential, and it pays off, because we're so caught up in the time thing. If I am centered, then everything around me begins to get quiet and centered. If I enter into the chaos and the anxiety, I might as well hang it up because it just multiplies and goes out of control.

When you hold this calmness, you hold it not only for yourself and the family but also for your colleagues around you. They are all affected by it. They feel it when you walk into a nurse's station.

We are all so connected. I don't want to speak as if I walk on water. When you walk on water, of course, you sink. I can't talk about suffering and compassion without speaking of rage.

Michael: Rage?

Katherine: Rage. I'll be working with someone I feel connected to and it's all wrong. Not only are they dying but maybe they're in pain, or they're leaving children behind, or they're very much needed, or they are a young couple or they've got much living to do. Whatever the issues are, it feels wrong. There is certain suffering that has me cry to God, "What are you doing? What is this about?"

I allow myself to go into that place of rage. I do not deny it. I do not walk away from it. I watch myself fill up, and then there is that pivotal person who pushes me over the edge.

What I find myself doing, which I do not do in meditative prayer, is demanding certain things – demanding a miracle, demanding that this patient's pain be gone, heart-to-heart tantrums, discussions, demands with God.

What most amazes me about it is how often the prayer is answered. That is the place of mystery. We've been making changes in pain medication, for example, and getting nowhere, and there is suddenly a breakthrough. It's always impressive enough that I step back and take a deep breath.

What God most asks of us is that we be in relationship. It became clear to me that being in relationship means being free to speak what is in my heart. If my heart is full of rage or despair or joy, God asks me to go into relationship with whatever is there in the moment.

I also think he has a sense of humor, that he must find me quite charming when I am stamping my feet. I am the mother of young children, and there have been times when I've had to resist laughing at them, but there are also times when they have moved me into compassion.

I grew up believing God moved furniture, that he had this intricate way of being involved with everything. God is everywhere and God is good. Then I moved out of that way of seeing and recognized free will and that he was not involved with our daily movements.

What I have learned since is that God is very present to the everyday. When I think he knows every hair on my head, I feel this incredible sense of presence. Yes, I have free will, and yes, there are opportunities, but I also feel this incredible orchestration that allows me to be a corridor in a certain moment just when somebody needs me. Or I happen to ask a question of someone I've never asked before that happens to be the exact right question. You experience this sort of thing so often that you begin to say, "This is bigger than my intuition, bigger than coincidence."

I experience this as orchestration. There are wonderful patterns that God is creating. Of course we get to walk away. We get to be blind and not see, or we get to be wide awake, in touch, showing up exactly where we need to be – these ripples in our lives and those around us.

Michael: You speak now as a Catholic. Miracles and Presence. I think about my own Catholic childhood and learning so young about the frailty of the flesh.

Katherine: As a Catholic I think of every year, as a child, having ashes placed on my forehead before Easter – the mystery of that. As a child you don't really understand it. It's very solemn, there is this dark smudge on your forehead, but I'm grateful for that tradition because our culture so much avoids that lament. And so I think how it was, at age seventeen volunteering in a veteran's hospital, watching these Vietnam vets come back, sometimes with no arms or no legs. I was so full of life and beginnings and potential in contrast to this manmade destruction. For whatever reason, I was able to bear witness to death and the frailty of being human.

Like you, I witnessed Christ on the cross, absolute suffering, from the time I was a young child. This image was not only an image of suffering but also of overcoming this suffering. Redemption. The full cycle.

Growing up in the East, we experienced the death in winter and the fullness of spring that very much becomes the foundation of your life repeated over and over again.

There is no doubt in my mind – forget my religious upbringing, forget all those traditions – I know from being with the dying that there is a soul, that there is a spirit, and that when that body shuts down spirit is released.

There is the physical frailty, the physical destruction, all of that which can be horrific and takes our breath away, balanced the whole time with knowing that this soul gets to be borne out of this body. Death is an act of birth.

What is intolerable is suffering inflicted by other people. That's where I go over the edge. If I find a patient who is being neglected, for example, through bad pain management and is dying miserably when it could have been a good death – peaceful – therein lies my despair. When I come into a situation where a family's needs have been disregarded, where someone didn't understand the importance of a tradition, therein lies my despair.

27

The Serenity Prayer and the Three Faces of Living Compassion

"God grant me the serenity to accept the things I cannot change, the courage to change the things I can, and the wisdom to know the difference."

The theologian Reinhold Neibuhr intoned this prayer at the end of the sermon on practical Christianity.

Living the serenity prayer shaves away the ego that refuses to accept what cannot be changed. The refusal to look life – and death – in the eye obscures the broadness that makes living compassion possible.

The other side of that ego is the fear to change the things that can be changed. This is the fierce edge of compassion that is so often what the elders speak of in this book.

Both the refusal to accept and the fear of stepping forth are about refusing to be present. Presence is the only place that living compassion can happen. When I was talking to my friend Carolyn Raffensperger about the wisdom to know the difference, she elaborated with the courage to bear witness.

Bearing witness pervades all of the prayer and in fact is the presence of compassion behind acceptance, the direct compassionate act and wisdom/discernment. Bearing witness accompanies all of our "successes" and "failures" in learning the craft of compassion.

Mrs. Shore was no less than 105 years old with a complex cardiac history and senile dementia. She had been incontinent of urine and stool and was pleasantly and perpetually confused. I had the honor of informing her that she was a woman.

"Oh, I'm so glad to hear about that!"

The shift was crazy busy. I was aware from the chart that her family wanted her not to be revived should she have a cardiac arrest. I could also see that her doctor had not signed the required "do not resuscitate" order. I also knew she was scheduled to have a central line wormed into her heart midmorning so she could have IV access that her skinny, bruised arms had tired of.

With some effort I finally connected with an intern before I left work in the morning. She agreed that Mrs. Shore could easily have a cardiac arrest and would make a point of having her primary physicians sign the DNR order before the insertion of the cardiac cath.

Living compassion with Mrs. Shore: to accept what I could not change – the simple reality of mortality and death.

Genpo Roshi, the Zen teacher, speaks of the yin and the yang faces of compassion, though he's clear that yin and yang are not about female and male gender. The serenity of accepting what cannot be changed is yin compassion. It is imaged as Kwan Yin, sometimes called the female Buddha. *Tonglen* is the practice – inhaling the suffering that is before one and exhaling lovingkindness. The soul expands as it drops denial and is quietly and reliably unafraid.

The keyword for the yin way of living compassion is "embrace." With Mrs. Shore, yin compassion was basking in the pleasure of our open and silly conversation and the joy in her discovery of her ancient womanly self. The embrace of yin is priceless. Spacious and free.

The effort to "change what I could" was disentangling Mrs. Shore from layers of *undecided decisions*. If the right signature was not in the right place, extreme measures of resuscitation would be initiated whatever the family's desires.

The courage to change the things that can be changed is yang compassion. It is imaged as Manjusri who bears the sword that cuts through the delusion of separateness. Manjusri's way of living compassion is no nonsense and forthright, sometimes the tough love that pierces through the organized lovelessness we face everyday. The sword is awakened when defending those who cannot defend themselves.

· I was aware of the yang aspect of living compassion when I could feel my whole self mobilize as I scanned her chart and put to the particulars together. Her cardiac history, the imminent heart catheterization, the unsigned DNR order, her dementia that made it impossible for her to advocate for herself and her family's wishes. "Mobilize" is the key word for the yang way of living compassion.

The wisdom to know the difference between what could and could not be changed rested in bearing witness, and bearing witness rested in the effortless mindfulness of living compassion.

My friend Peter Levitt, a Buddhist practitioner, once asked Kwong Roshi of the Sonoma Mountain Zen Center, why is it that the images of Kwan Yin are so sweet and warm while the images of Manjusri with his sword ready to strike show him terrifying in his ferocity. Kwong Roshi responded, "Oh you must understand Manjusri's sword cuts through delusion."

"So the heart of Kwan Yin and the sword of Manjusri are the same?" said Peter.

"Exactly."

Conclusion: The Best You Can Ever Do

This book is an extended meditation on the epigraphs at the beginning, so it is right that the conclusion folds back to those insights.

William Blake said: "We are put on earth but a little space / That we might learn to bear the beams of love."

The edge of this life – its preciousness, its peculiarity, its radiant finitude – is the precise place we meet another's sorrow with our sorrow, another's joy with our joy. This is a blessed life's work, the circumstance that transforms us. A critical understanding throughout is that every gesture of kindness to another is simultaneously a gesture toward one's own awakening.

In living compassion we realize that the other is our self.

So in this little space of our little life we hasten slowly, act impeccably, mindful of the self we share with another.

The Zen teacher Cheri Huber captures the spirit of this exactly:

"Love as much as you can from where you are with what you've got. That's the best you can ever do. Remember, it's the process, not the content that counts."

The process is the moment by moment practice of learning what it means to practice compassion for ourselves and others in a world of suffering. We will fail and we will forgive our failures but in truth "success" and "failure" do not describe the process we are in.

Everything instructs the heart.

Everything.

Compassion toward the self for falling short delivers directly to compassion for others because no one is unfamiliar with the sense of failure.

The West African novelist Ama Ata Aidoo says "work is love made visible" and the registered nurse, Carolyn Fink, writes of the epiphany of that visible love:

"In the middle of nursing duties and dirty beds and bloody bandages there is magic. Where there is pain and fear and loneliness, there are miracles. In the small hours of the night when there are dying and dark things, there is light."

One walks three steps toward the light and then steps into it.

Steps One and Two: unimpeded in compassion toward yourself, you learn to be without obstacle in compassion toward another.

Step Three follows effortlessly. Radical empathy – joined at the root with another you know that the face of the beloved is also your face. You move with a transparent familiarity with the circumstances of being human.

And finally you come to Step Four, this light, this paradigm shift.

The *mysterium* of living compassion is in this light and in this light, love is made visible.

T.S. Eliot writes:

> *We shall never cease from exploration*
> *And the end of all our exploring*
> *Will be to arrive where we started*
> *And know the place for the first time.*

And so it is with the craft of compassion, for we forever return to loving this peculiar self made in God's image and love him or her unconditionally. True love does not divide self from other and the mandate of living love sees no one unworthy of love. Living compassion *is* loving the self and the other selflessly.

If I have learned anything from my years of labor in the salt mines of western medicine it's that the opportunity to love is always now, the place, this very place. From now and from exactly where you are – withhold nothing. Follow the contours of this arc (of your heart) – loving yourself and daring to love all you meet, dare even to live compassion – then the craft of generosity will become the vibrant truth that you live for.

Michael Ortiz Hill is a registered nurse, a Buddhist practitioner, and an initiated medicine man with tribal people of Zimbabwe. The core of his spiritual practice has been the refinement and activity of compassion. He is the author of *Dreaming the End of the World: Apocalypse as a Rite of Passage*; *Twin from Another Tribe: The Story of Two Shamanic Healers in Africa and North America*; and *The Village of the Water Spirits: The Dreams of African-Americans* (both books with Mandaza Kandemwa). Michael gives workshops on the Craft of Compassion. His website is www.gatheringin.com He lives in Topanga, California with his wife, Deena Metzger.

References:

Glaser, Aura, *Call To Compassion: Bringing Buddhist Practices Of The Heart Into The Soul Of Psychology*, Weiser, 2005

Ladner, Ph.D., Lorne, *The Art of Compassion, Discovering the Practice of Happiness in the Meeting of Buddhism and Psychology*, Harper Collins, 2004.

Makransky, John, *Awakening Through Love: Unveiling Your Deep Goodness*, Wisdom Publications, 2007.

Smith, Zadie, "Always Another Word," Readings, *Harper's Magazine*, January 2009.

Watson, Ph.D., RN, Jean, *Nursing: The Philosophy and Science of Caring*, University Press of Colorado, 1991.